The Collected Writings of

Robert J. Neborsky, MD

The Collected Writings of
Robert J. Neborsky, MD

Unlocking Press
DEL MAR, CALIFORNIA

Tasora

Published by
Unlocking Press
317 Fourteenth Street
Del Mar, CA 92014

Printed in the United States of America on acid-free paper

ISBN-13: 978-1-934690-24-6

Cover design by Joanna Neborsky
Interior text design by BookMobile Design and Publishing Services

To order additional copies of this book please contact:
Tasora Books
5120 Cedar Lake Road
Minneapolis, MN 55416
(952) 345-4488
Distributed by Itasca Books

To Sandra

a wonderful partner whose
love and support made this work possible

Table of Contents

Foreword

I was introduced to my colleague Josette ten Have-de Labije at the first International Experiential Dynamic Therapy Association conference held in Milan, Italy in 2001, where she presented the video tape of her case "The War-Traumatized Patient." The video took my breath away. Since that time, I have enjoyed many occasions to marvel at the purity, brilliance, and creativity of her technique. In the 1990s she was a student of Habib Davanloo, with whom I studied in the early 1980s. We both struggled to learn his technique. At that time he had not systematized his teaching; my learning was mostly by imitation, as well as an attempt to read between the lines of his clinical brilliance. I completed my Core Training in 1986 and Dr. Davanloo and I went our separate ways.

In 1994, after an interlude of silence, Dr. Davanloo asked me to discuss his cases at UCLA in a conference sponsored by the Lifespan Learning Institute. As a result of that conference, I wrote the first article in Volume I, *Les Misérables: A Metapsychologic Analysis,* which was published in the now-defunct *International Journal of Short-Term Dynamic Psychotherapy,* edited by Davanloo. It was my attempt to apply his concept of the superego and ego to a work of literature. Once I started looking at patients and pathology through the lens that he taught me, a new world of clinical possibilities opened up, which led me to write "The Role of the Sibling in the Unconscious." Next I authored a paper based on the case I presented at the Milan Conference where I had met Josette (*Perinatal Trauma, Anxiety and Resistance against Emotional Closeness–The Song of Bernadette,* 2002). Looking back I can see these writings as my pre-conscious attempts to master Davanloo's thinking. I had already written many chapters in the multi-author book *Short-term Therapy for Long-Term Change* (WW Norton, 2001), which detailed my initial understanding of his work. I speculated in that book that attachment trauma was the underlying basis of ego-superego difficulties—not unresolved oedipal complexes. Today I remain convinced.

During the time I spent in LA, I also served as medical director for Marion and Mathew Solomon's continuing education organization, The Lifespan Learning Institute. During my tenure I became intrigued by both attachment theory and affective neuroscience. At the Institute I met Mary Main, Erik Hesse, Daniel Siegel, Allan Shore, Dan Stern, T. Berry Brazelton, Ed Tronick, Jaak Panksepp, Steve Porges, and many others. In these scientists and clinicians I observed first-rate minds struggling to integrate the science of our time with psychotherapy.

In 2002, another shift occurred in my approach. I enjoyed the privilege of presenting with Mary Main at a UCSD-sponsored conference in San Diego, where I saw her work on disorganized attachment. Next I took the Adult Attachment Interview training with Don Pedersen in London. Their teachings fit perfectly with my theory; I began to work on clinical research with Mary Main and Erik Hesse. The remainder of the articles in Volume 1, from 2003 to 2009, expands on this area of clinical application and experimentation.

Back in 2001, I began to teach at conferences that Josette ten Have-de Labije sponsored in Europe and summer schools throughout the world. Eventually she invited me to be guest editor of the Dutch Association's *Ad Hoc Bulletin of Short-Term Dynamic Psychotherapy: Practice and Theory.* This was the seminal event that consolidated our cooperation and mutual respect. We began to edit each other's publications and to understand each other's thinking. In her I discovered the one person who could follow Davanloo's way of thinking just as well as the man himself. As the reader will discover, Josette has a highly developed systematic mind. She has organized Davanloo's therapeutic approach to reach the unconscious in a series of red and green traffic lights that allow students to appreciate and apply Davanloo's clinical genius. This body of work is an extraordinary feat and needs to be shared with a larger audience. Hers is an intellectual accomplishment that supercedes anything that I have been able to accomplish, despite my close working relationship with Davanloo. She has organized her volume not in a chronological order, but in an order to help the reader follow the logical progression of why ISTDP should be practiced the way she suggests.

Josette, a registered psychotherapist and clinical psychologist, is Dutch by birth. She came to be Davanloo's student when he started to give a core-training in the Netherlands. She started her professional career at the department of neuro- and psychophysiology at the Free University of Brussels (Belgium). After three years she switched to psychotherapy. She is trained as a cognitive and behavior therapist (individuals and groups), a couples' therapist, a psychodynamic psychotherapist, and a psychodynamic group psychotherapist. She wrote several articles on the autonomy problems of women, a self-help book on fear of flying (both in Dutch); she edited a book on cancer research and she organized several international conferences. She clearly understands the structured approach and learning theory principles which Davanloo's therapy uses to create symptom and character change. My observation of her work has inspired me to bestow on her the title "The Rembrandt of the Superego." She is an artist who paints a portrait of the patient's disturbed attachment-based punitive superego with a beauty and precision exemplified by Rembrandt's portraits of Dutch citizens.

The educational goal of these two volumes is to illustrate the way two clinicians have struggled to decode Davanloo's brilliant method. The reader will see the interaction of two dedicated minds grappling with the incredibly difficult task of learning, teaching, and practicing Intensive Short-Term Dynamic Psychotherapy. Given the complexity of the human psyche, there is no task as daunting as attempting to treat a patient in depth in psychotherapy in as short a period of time as possible. I hope you will gain new appreciation for the magnitude of the challenge.

Robert J. Neborsky, MD
March 2010
Del Mar, California

Les Misérables by Victor-Marie Hugo

A Metapsychological Analysis

Both the novel and the opera *Les Misérables* have enjoyed worldwide success. The novel by Victor Hugo was first published in 1862. Hugo by the age of thirty was a recognized master of the arts of poetry, drama, and fiction. He was a political figure as well, and in 1851, he was banished to the Channel Isle of Guernsey for opposing Louis Napoleon's coup. During his twenty-year exile, he wrote a number of novels, the most notable of which, was the masterpiece *Les Misérables.* Following his death in Paris in 1885, his greatness was recognized by the French people as he was placed in state beneath the Arc de Triumph. He was later buried in Pantheon among France's greatest men.

The idea of turning *Les Misérables* into a musical came to Alain Boublil one evening in 1979 during a visit to London. He collaborated with Claude-Michael Schonberg in which they transformed the 1,500 page book into an opera libretto of three acts, seven tableaux. *Les Misérables* opened at the Palais des Sports in Paris in September of 1980. It was directed by Robert Osein. During its three-month season, the first production was seen by over a million people. In 1982, Cameron Mackintosh invited Claude-Michael Schonberg, Alain Boublil, Trevor Nunn, John Caird, James Fenton to rework an English version of the musical (Boublil, 1986). Herbert Kretzmer joined the group to create English counterparts of the original French lyrics as well as adding new lyrics, especially for the English production. It opened at the Barbican Theatre on October 8, 1985, and was transferred on December 4 of that year to the Palace Theatre for an enormously successful run. The Broadway production opened to equal success on March 12, 1987, and like Hugo's original book reached a worldwide public. It was awarded the 1987 Musical Cast Album and won the 1987 Tony Award for best musical.

The immense popularity of the novel as well as the opera fascinates me because the story line is exceedingly complex as well as contrived. Furthermore, something within the story line creates a powerful emotional response in its audiences. The great literary critic Norman Holland and others have offered a psychoanalytic theory of the way a work of art affects the audience (Holland, 1968). Holland professes that in reading or watching a work of art, a dream is "dreamed for us, which we then introject" [p. 89]. He goes on to state "a literary work embodies a specific mental process, the transformation of a normally unconscious fantasy toward conscious, intellectual meaning." I interpret his work to mean that great works of art capture for us great unconscious themes that are cleverly disguised to escape our "dream censor" and allow the viewer to gain closer access to his subconscious, giving a deep emotional response.

Therefore, the purpose of this paper is to offer a new psychoanalytic interpretation to explain the universal emotional response to this particular artistic creation. At a recent Los Angeles symposium where I discussed a technical analysis of the clinical tapes presented by Dr. Habib Davanloo, it occurred to me as I listened the next day to a recording of *Les Misérables* that the main character, Jean Valjean, struggles with a neurotic problem much like those patients I discussed in Dr. Davanloo's tapes (Davanloo, 1994). Many works of art are interpreted using psychoanalytic literary theory (Margo, 1992), but only one other work of art, *King Lear,* is studied *through* Dr. Davanloo's revolutionary metapsychologic theory (Margo, 1992). In his paper on *King Lear,* Dr. Margo begins this process when he compares the audience's reaction to the dramatic portrayal of the tragic figure of Lear to the experience one gets viewing the Trial Model of Therapy on one of Davanloo's tapes. Clearly, Davanloo's technique greatly enriches our profession's understanding of human neurosis, and secondarily, the application of his meta-psychology now begins to unlock our understanding of works of art (Davanloo, 1990).

I will now attempt to explain how such a confusing, intricate story, set in the post-Bonaparte restoration, has such Universal appeal. The opera is true to the basic story line of the novel; so, for the modern reader, I will direct my analysis mainly to the opera. For maximum enjoyment of this paper I suggest the readers listen to a recorded version of *Les Misérables* before and after reading this analysis. My psychologic analysis of the structure of the story reveals three separate phases to this work: Suffering, Transformation, and Restoration. These phases are commented on in the italicized comments interspersed into the story line.

Suffering: The First Act

The action begins in 1815 when Jean Valjean, imprisoned for twenty-plus years for "the theft of a loaf of bread" is released with the stigma of the yellow card identifying him as an ex-convict. We see an expressionistic picture of beaten men marching timelessly in a neverending circle. The chorus sings:

Look down, look down . . .
Don't look em in the eye
Look down, look down
You're here until you die.
The sun is strong, it's hot as hell below

Look down, look
down It's twenty
years to go . . .
• • •
How long before you let me die?
Look down, look down
You'll always be a slave

The tone is set for the audience: we see Jean Valjean as a man locked in existential misery. He is depressed, oppressed, bitter, and trapped in a maze of perpetual self-punishment from which there is no apparent escape. We are informed that his prison sentence was so long because he unsuccessfully attempted to escape three times. In his forty-eighth-year of life, which should be the peak of mid-life creativity, we see instead a disenfranchised victim wandering in rural France, ostracized from respectable society.

He is finally, through the mercy of the Bishop of Digne, given lodging, food, and emotional support. Jean Valjean is touched for the first time, in who knows how many years, by the humanitarian love of the Bishop who welcomes him in his home and hearth despite Jean Valjean's criminal record. The antihero, however, is consumed by his own rage and wishes for vengeance against those who have wronged him so he steals the Bishop's Sacramental silver candlesticks. Jean Valjean flees in the night like the thief that he is, and as is the pattern, of his neurosis, he is caught and expects to receive more self-induced punishment. He is about to be returned to prison when the Bishop intercedes on behalf of Jean Valjean. The Bishop lies to the Gendarmes and tells them that the stolen silver was actually a gift. Privately, he entreats Jean Valjean to take the silver, sell it, build a new life based on good works and love of humanity in return for the Bishop's kindness. Valjean is touched, and vows to start his life anew.

The scene shifts and eight years have passed. The audience now sees a bleak picture of the hopeless existence of the working class in early 19th-century France. The chorus sings:

At the end of the day you're another day older
And that's all you can say for the life of the poor
At the end of the day you're another day colder
And that's all you can say for the life of the poor
It's a struggle—it's a war—and there's nothing that anyone's giving.
One more day standing about,
what is it for?
One less day to be living
One day nearer to dying.

It is now 1823 and Valjean, having broken his parole and changed his name to Monsieur Madeleine, has become both a factory owner and the mayor of the town. However, Valjean is still crippled by subconscious motives and superego destruction, and thus tragedy unfolds. The music communicates the swirling tragic forces lurking in and around Jean Valjean.

One of his factory workers, Fantine, has a secret illegitimate child. When the other women employees discover this, they demand Fantine be exiled. Jean Valjean's foreman throws her out *(abandonment)* to a life of poverty and depravity when she rejects his sexual advances.

> As they tear your hope apart, as they turn your dream to shame.
> He slept a summer by my side. He filled my days with endless
> wonder. He took my childhood in his stride.
> But he was gone when autumn came . . .
>
> I had a dream my life would be so different from this hell I'm living;
> so different from what it seemed.
> Now life has killed the dream I dreamed.

Valjean is a man of great physical strength and he rescues a man pinned down by a runaway cart. Javert observes this act of great physical strength, reminding him of a convict who could lift great weights "like a jack knife"—the parole breaker he has been tracking for years. Javert is the local Constable who is Valjean's nemesis. We are told Javert was born and raised in the same squalor as Valjean; but he, Javert, respects THE LAW. Therefore, he will hunt, stalk and punish Valjean until he, too, learns to respect THE LAW, like Javert.

> There, out in the darkness, a fugitive running, fallen from grace.
> God, be my witness. I shall never yield till we come face to face. He
> knows his way in the dark, but mine is the way of the Lord. And if
> they fall as Lucifer fell, the flame, the sword!
> And so it has been and so it is written on the doorways to Paradise,
> that those who falter and those who fall must pay the price.

Fantine worked at the factory to support her lovely illegitimate child, Cosette, whom she naively left in the care of two psychopathic inn-keepers, Monsieur and Madame Thenardier. Desperate for money to pay for Cosette's care (she was relentlessly scammed for money by Thenardier with one false story about Cosette after another), Fantine becomes a prostitute, sells her hair, her teeth (in the novel), and her belongings out of desperation. Javert arrests Fantine for fighting with an abusive customer but Valjean intercedes on her behalf. He discovers Fantine is dying from malnutrition and disease.

Meanwhile, Valjean has discovered an innocent man in Paris has been accused via mistaken identity of being the escapee 24601. *In an act of martyrdom*, Valjean confesses his true identity before the court and Javert in order to save the accused innocent.

Can I conceal myself forever more?
Pretend I'm not the man I was before?
And must my name until I die be no
more than an alibi? . . . Who am I? I'm
Jean Valjean!
Who am I? 24601!

He leaves the court, returns to Fantine's bedside, and promises the dying Fantine to find and look after her daughter Cosette. Javert arrives to arrest him, but Valjean escapes. Valjean rescues Cosette, recognizes the deplorable way she is treated by the Thenardiers, but he does nothing to avenge her and Fantine. He meekly ransoms her from their bondage and abuse.

As a work of art, this action makes little sense until we approach the story from a metapsychologic point of view. Jean Valjean is archetypal man. He carries with him guilt from unconscious rage and sadistic impulses from his own childhood trauma. He, like all neurotics, is relentlessly punished by the repetition compulsion forces, emanating from his own superego. Javert is the symbolic representation of Jean Valjean's superego. Despite Jean Valjean's attempts by his conscious ego to deny, rationalize, and undo, he is destined for self-destruction unless he enters his own subconscious to cleanse the structure of his neurosis.

Hence the dramatic appearance of Fantine, a woman placed on the fringes of society for having born a child out of wedlock. Fantine suffers horribly. She has naively left her child in the care of the psychopathic Thenardiers, who exploit both Fantine for money and Cosette for child labor. They also abuse the child.

The convoluted story finally begins to demonstrate psychologic meaning. Fantine represents Jean Valjean's mother. She is the mother of the past who neglected him, who inadequately provided for him and allowed him to be exposed to trauma. Jean Valjean's most unforgivable "sin" is his unconscious sadistic and murderous rage at his mother. The Thenardiers are the embodiment of Jean Valjean's unconscious psychopathic impulses and feelings. Cosette is the innocent Child, the tableau rosa that once was Jean Valjean.

The Second Act: Transformation

It is now 1832; the scene is Paris nine years later. There is great unrest in the city because a popular leader, General Lamarque, is about to die. The poor are tired, hungry, angry and spoiling for a fight. The Thenardiers are now in Paris with their two children, Gavroche and Eponine. These are the same children who benefited from Fantine's money and exploited Cosette along with their parents. They are part of the begging, thievery, and debauchery of 1832 Paris.

A new character appears by the name of Marius who is a young penniless lawyer and naive political idealist. Valjean and Cosette have lived in hiding under assumed identities in Paris for the past nine years. Marius has seen Cosette on walks with her doting, aging "father" Jean Valjean. He has fallen head over heels in love with her. Cosette, unbeknownst to Marius, has fallen equally in love with him. Marius however cannot be united with Cosette because he believes she has left the country. He becomes desperately depressed and joins his friend Enjolras in a spontaneous student rebellion against the current government.

> Do you hear the people singing the song
> of angry men? It is the music of people
> who will not be slaves again!
> When the beating of your heart echoes the beating of
> the drums, there is a life when tomorrow comes.
> Will you join in our crusade? . . .
> Will you stand up and take our chance?
> The blood of the martyrs will water the
> meadows of France! Do you hear the people
> singing the song of angry men?
> It is the music of a people who will not be slaves again!

The rebellion is part political and part a flash riot of angry peasants. The students hope to ignite a serious uprising through their own martyrdom. Marius and the students confront the forces of social oppression at the infamous and highly symbolic barricade.

Through Marius's angry rebellion, Jean Valjean can be set free from the slavery that is the consequence of his neurosis.

In the action, Javert sneaks behind the barricade in order to spy for THE LAW. Jean Valjean also sneaks behind the barricade as well but his motive is to rescue Marius so that he and Cosette can unite and marry. Jean Valjean is greeted by the rebels as a great hero for sneaking by the French guard. The two young Thenardiers, Eponine and Gavroche, are both killed by the French Militia. Eponine dies while acting out of love for Marius to send a message to Cosette. Gavroche dies honorably trying to procure ammunition for the rebels.

Their deaths symbolize the early transformation of the deeply repressed unconscious sadistic impulses towards mother and siblings within Jean Valjean as he approaches the unlocking of his unconscious.

Red, the blood of angry men, Black, the
night that ends at last Red, I feel my
soul on fire, Black, I feel my world if
she's not there Red, the colour of desire,
Black, the colour of despair
Red, the blood of angry men, Black, the dark of ages past

There is now no turning back as the forces of mutilation and death are unleashed. Jean Valjean's entrance into his own subconscious is now unavoidable. Javert is captured by Enjolras and Jean Valjean is given the reward of being allowed to execute Javert in the name of the revolution. Despite the cruelty, despite the oppression, despite Javert's brutal stalking, Jean Valjean compassionately releases Javert to his own forces [much like the Bishop did for Jean Valjean]. He leaves, but all is lost: everyone is killed in the holocaust which ensues. The militia overwhelms the barricade and slaughters the rebels.

Beyond the barricade is there a world you'd love to see? Then join the fight that would give you the right to be free!

Symbolically the barricade represents the boundary between conscious and subconscious, between psychopathic rage and relentless self punishment. It now becomes apparent that the revolution represents the personal crisis which occurs in midlife or intensive psychotherapy when one encounters the unconscious rage that has produced a life of unfulfilled potentiality. Marius is Jean Valjean's alter ego. Marius is confronting in his youth the forces of his oppression so that Jean Valjean can be restored to wholeness and thereby freed from his own self-imposed isolation from heterosexual love.

Somehow Jean Valjean survives the assault by the Militia and rescues the nearly mortally wounded Marius. The only escape route from certain death is through the sewers of Paris. In one of the great scenes of Western literature, Jean Valjean carries Marius on his back through the fetid slime of the sewer.

Bring him home, bring him home, bring him home.
He is like the son I might have known if God had granted me a son.
The summers die one by one. How soon they fly on and on. And
I am old and will be gone. Bring him peace bring him joy. He is
young, he is only a boy.

In a bizarre coincidence Jean Valjean encounters Thenardier who is scavenging gold from the bodies of Marius's dead comrades.

In the deepest layer of the "unconscious," Jean Valjean encounters, face to face, his disavowed counterpart, Thenardier. After this encounter with his own nightmarish cannibalistic counterpart, purification has occurred. Marius and Jean Valjean emerge from the sewer of the subconscious and return to life.

The next scene shows Marius deep in mourning for his comrades who died in combat. The scene with the haunting elegy "Empty chairs, empty tables" shows us his pain.

> There's a grief that can't be spoken. There's a pain that goes on and on. Empty chairs at empty tables, now my friends are dead and gone. Here they talked on revolution. Here it was they lit the flame . . . There's a grief that can't be spoken There's a pain that goes on and on.

> *Pathologic bereavement (for Jean Valjean) is now acute grief in Marius. Like all patients who suffer the extreme range of trauma, Jean Valjean/ Marius experiences the deepest level of emotional pain as he grieves his own loss along with the guilt laden feelings about corpses of those he has sadistically mutilated in his own Unconscious.*

Restoration

Marius takes Cosette from Jean Valjean and Valjean's health wanes. He is now ready for welcome death as his lovely ward Cosette is separated from him and in the arms of Marius. He is melancholic and frail.

> *The character Jean Valjean must die since through the transformation, he no longer exists except as a shell. In the law of the Unconscious when a loved object is decathected it results in the dissolution (death) of that object. Jean Valjean's unconscious marriage to Fantine is dissolved. He is now free to die.*

Restoration is now underway. Javert, the superego of relentless punishment, dies at his own hand because of the crisis he faced when he was spared by Jean Valjean. He sings

> How can I allow this man to hold dominion over me?
> I should have perished by his hand
> Can this man be forgiven? Can his crime be reprieved? Must I now begin to doubt? The world I have known is lost in a shadow
> From the world of Jean Valjean there is no where I can turn.
> There is no way I can go on . . .

and then throws himself into the most lethal part of the Seine.

> *Once the hated criminal, Valjean, treated Javert with love, once Valjean emerged into the truth of his own subconscious, the superego as it always*

does, transforms into a kind, benevolent, supportive structure. The self-abusive Superego is fueled by the energy of Unconscious murderous range and sadism. So, Jean Valjean has completed the transformation from Thenardiers (UNCS) through Gavroche and Eponine (PRECS) to Marius and Cosette (CS). He is now a whole human being. Marius and Cosette are married. (Figure 1).

Mind	*Process*	*Character*		*Scene*	*Metapsychologic Event*
Spiritual	**Transformation**	Jean Valjean and Fantine		Heaven	Loving Superego Freed
Conscious	**Birth of New Self**	Marius and Cosette's		Marriage	Acceptance of Love by Ego
Preconscious	**Restoration**	Javert dies		Javert's Suicide	Death of Punitive Superego
	Mourning	Jean Valjean		Empty Tables	Decathexis of past love objects
	Rebellion Against Old Order	Gavroche	Eponine	The Barricade	Separation of ego from superego
Unconscious	**Revenge Relinquished**	Jean Valjean rescues Marius		The Sewer	Working through Retaliatory Rage
	Sadism and Masochism	Thenardier	Mme Thenardier	The Sewer	

Figure 1. The metapsychologic progression of *Les Misérables*

Jean Valjean appears dying. The Thenardiers appear at the wedding feast but this time they are banished forever by a whole, assertive Marius, *symbolically ending the domination of Jean Valjean's personality.*

Jean Valjean dies and Marius and Cosette are unified in the harmonic oneness of their intimacy, closeness, and sexuality with no contamination by the destructive forces of the ever-lurking superego. They are not tragically destined for destruction like Jean Valjean and Fantine were.

In the moving ending, Fantine and Jean Valjean are reunited in heaven, removed from this world where they suffered so much pain. They look at Marius and Cosette who are both whole and restored. Fantine sings

> Come with me where chains will never bind you
> Where your dreams are at last behind you
> Remember the words once spoken,
> To love another person is to see the face of God
>
> *Jean Valjean [nee: Marius] can now love a female in a whole and complete way because the murderer within him has decathected his repressed rage toward the mother of abuse and abandonment.*

Great artists have always been able to capture the subtleties of the human psyche. Rarely, however, does an artist ever capture the full picture of the Unconscious in such a disguised way. Without a doubt, Victor Hugo magically captures the essence of human neurosis in his masterpiece, *Les Misérables.* It is my assertion that this complex and somewhat idiosyncratic story resonates with the deepest layers of the Unconscious Mind. This, according to Holland's model of art as a "waking dream," explains the universal popularity of this story and opera.

On a more personal level, my attempt to apply Davanloo's Metapsychology to a great work of Western fiction as well as an enormously popular modern opera has given me great pleasure. Rather than simply listening and/or watching a performance (or reading a novel), the process has actually become a therapeutic working through of my own subconscious emotion. It is my hope, in writing this paper, that I can extend this wondrous experience to other interested practitioners of Davanloo's method of psychoanalysis.

BIBLIOGRAPHY

Boublil, A., Schonberg, C. & Kretzmer, H. (1986). *Les Misérables, the Musical Sensation.* Alain Boublil Music Ltd.

Davanloo, H. (1994). *Symposium in Intensive Short-Term Dynamic Psychotherapy.* Los Angeles, CA.

Davanloo, H. (1990). *Unlocking the Unconscious.* Chichester, John Wiley and Sons.

Holland, N. (1968). *The Dynamics of Literary Response.* Oxford University Press.

Hugo, V. (1862). *Les Misérables.*

Margo, G. (1992). "Pathways to the Unconscious: A Parallel Analysis of Shakespeare's *King Lear* and Davanloo's Central Dynamic Sequence." *International Journal of Short-Term Psychotherapy*, 7, 199–210.

Reprinted with permission of publisher J. Wiley and author, *International Journal of Short-Term Dynamic Psychotherapy*, pp. 222–225, 1990.

The Role of the Sibling in the Unconscious

Sibling jealousy, or *sibling rivalry,* is a significant issue in family relationships. Throughout the contemporary world, healthy as well as "dysfunctional" families find themselves dealing with children arguing about *who gets to go to bed later, who has the bigger piece of cake,* and *who gets to push the button in the elevator!* (Recognize the anguished cry, *it's not fair*?) Certainly, these are benign forms of sibling rivalry, but sibling issues are essential to understanding growth and development, as well as the workings of the unconscious.

The Bible describes more extreme examples of sibling discontent. After Adam and Eve were *banished* from the Garden of Eden, they entered a phase, what we today term a "committed relationship." Before long, Eve gave birth to Cain, a strapping young boy. Another son, Abel, was born soon after. Cain, it appears, was not everyone's favorite fellow. Scholars tell us he was moody and prone to anger. Cain not only resented having to sacrifice to G-d, but was angrier still that G-d was displeased with his attitude. *Perhaps his negative character was the result of Eve being depressed and unable to supply a loving environment. Was she depressed because of her banishment from the Garden of Eden? Did this contribute to Cain's personality disorder?*

After the birth of her second child, Eve appears to have recovered from depression. Abel is described as a happy child—free-spirited, bearing a positive disposition. *It looks like Abel's Pre-Oedipal experience was not only sufficient, but comfortable.* In contrast to Cain, he sacrificed to G-d willingly and with joy.

This only made matters worse for Cain. He was furious that he did not have the respect that his brother enjoyed. Jealousy and rage overcame any sense of reason, and he killed his own brother. *The ultimate in sibling rivalry ends in murder.*

When G-d inquired about Abel, Cain belligerently cried: "Am I my brother's keeper?" G-d knew that Cain was not telling the truth. "The blood of your brother cries out to me from the ground. Because of that, the earth that drinks the bloodshed by your hand shall forever curse you. When you till the soil it will not yield its crops for you: from this day you will be a wanderer and fugitive throughout the land." Thus we have, so soon after the creation of man, a heinous crime—fratricide. *It highlights the magnitude of sibling rivalry in the universality of human experience.*

The thread of sibling rivalry surfaces in other Bible stories. Abraham's son, Jacob, steals his father's last blessing from his older brother Esau, and thus must leave home. Joseph, another victim of fraternal jealousy resulting from his father's obvious partiality, is sold into slavery by his own brothers.

There are countless references that help us understand the power of the unconscious. Primitive societies have always struggled with aggressive behaviors within their community, as well as from other tribes. Sibling competition for paternal favor produced family tension when survival depended on ownership of land and water rights. This atmosphere allowed the murder of favored siblings by other siblings to take place. How better to develop a super-ego prohibition against the murder of a blood relative?

In today's modern world, I practice Intensive Short-Term Dynamic Psychotherapy. This therapy gives me a unique opportunity to examine sibling relationships in the unconscious of adult neurotic patients. For those unfamiliar with ISTDP, it is an accelerated analytic therapy in which ego and super-ego resistance are exhausted in the first few hours of treatment, and a unique phenomenon referred to as *the unconscious therapeutic alliance* occurs. In this state of mind, the unconscious often "holds on" to repressed sadistic impulses and feelings. The trained clinician recognizes these symptoms and can clearly determine the core patricidal, matricidal, and/or fratricidal emotions from the patients' dynamic past.

Traditionally, neurotic psychopathology is traced back to the Oedipus complex. The male child, for example, experiences the father as a rival for the primary nurturer/sexual object . . . his mother. The son, feeling excluded from the mother-child dyad, is enraged and experiences murderous impulses toward his rival . . . his own father. A subsequent sense of guilt (for the psychological murder of the father) is now present. In the best of circumstances, there is an adequate nurturing paternal bond, combined with good maternal boundaries, and the son is able to repress the Oedipal attraction for mother. Happily, he now develops a strong positive sense of masculine self, based on identification with the father. Latency gives quiescence to the intensity of Oedipal passion and an opportunity for father and son to further consolidate their identification through schoolwork, games and sports, as well as in everyday family life.

With the onset of adolescence and the resultant upsurge of the libido from the hormonal surge, sexuality again presents itself. In normal adolescent males, the sexual instinctual urges are now directed away from incestual objects and focus on girlfriends, movie stars, teachers, or magazine models. In normal adolescent male development, the pursuit of a non-incestual, nurturing/sexual relationship begins. Different subcultures within our society define how and when this unfolds, but the developmental task is the same . . . to separate from the primary nurturing/sexual objects and to replace them with a non-incestual selection.

At the same time, the father's role changes from that of *rival* to *buddy*. This helps define a role model the son either identifies with or rebels against as he begins to consolidate his identity. Also at this time, the peer group takes on significant importance. Social grouping takes place and complex issues relating to competition and cooperation are worked through successfully, or they create traumatic points of fixation. In some ways, this is the cauldron of sibling rivalry that all young people must master. They must find their social rank within the peer group and deal with the painful issues of popularity/unpopularity, achievement/failure, and selfishness/consideration for others.

Following adolescence, the final stage of separation occurs. The young adult can now successfully establish himself as an independent, self sufficient person with a role in a social system. Conversely, underlying neurotic and characterologic *unconscious* instincts will create reenactments in adult life. These reenactments are referred to as repetition compulsions.

Pre-Oedipal experience is a major factor in the development of neurotic psychopathology. In my practice, I have found that the greater the Pre-Oedipal trauma, the harsher the superego, resulting in *extreme* masochistic needs of the patient. My work confirms that the foundation of the super-ego is formed in the Pre-Oedipal stages of life. The appearance of a sibling in a compromised maternal child dyad forms early triangulation trauma that can pre-stage the relatively less toxic Oedipal triangulation. What occurs, again, is a severely sadistic unconscious organization of a particularly virulent nature. These patients frequently have markedly fragile ego organizations. They also have a proclivity for *acting out* . . . often abusing alcohol and drugs. The degree of self-destructive behavior directly correlates to the degree of unconscious sadism. And this, in turn, directly correlates to the depth of the trauma to the developing ego in the child.

Instinctual endowment obviously plays a role, but that is often hard to quantify. Suffice to say that over endowment of aggressive or libidinal instinct causes trauma as the child tries to work out his equilibrium with the environment. We now refer to him as *the difficult child.* These children present challenges to even the most empathetic parents. In this cluster, the children often have neuro-psychological deficits: short attention spans, impulse control difficulties, and/or hyperactive motor problems. *Each one of these characteristics is a potential contributory factor to adult neurosis.*

Oedipal Sibling Disturbance

Josh is a forty-five-year old emergency room physician who appears to be an excellent candidate for intensive short-term treatment: high functioning, with low resistance. He seeks treatment for episodic depression, along with severe marital disturbance. His wife often infuriates him to the threshold of near violence, and he is aware of the direct relationship between his rage and the depression that follows. He also complains of feeling distant and uninvolved in relating to his colleagues and patients. On a positive note, he has two children he loves deeply.

Family History

The father, a psychiatrist, is described as cold, distant and exploitative. Their relationship was estranged for many years. When his father died,

Josh was essentially disinherited, and the money was given to an endowed chair at the University.

The mother, extremely self-centered and difficult, is fiercely competitive with Josh's wife. On his wedding day, Josh remembers his mother vowing to destroy the marriage because *"she would not allow any woman come between me and my son."* After observing the dynamics of her in-laws, his wife totally disengaged from Josh's family. She suggested that he seek therapy. This was done in a very healthy and caring way.

Josh's mother and father divorced soon after he started medical school.

He has one sibling, a younger brother named David. David was an incredibly gifted child with a talent for language, music, mathematics and the dramatic arts. He was considered a prodigy. *In contrast, Josh was studious, shy, and reserved . . . a socially awkward child.* Years later, while in college, David developed schizophrenia. He now lives in a board and care facility on the East coast.

After Josh's father retired from his psychiatric practice, he told Josh that he would not take care of David any longer. He decided that David was to be solely Josh's responsibility. Suddenly, Josh was indeed, his brother's keeper.

Treatment

The therapy revealed a pathologic bereavement for his father. The father was a Hungarian refugee who had come to the United States to escape the Holocaust. Even though he was difficult to relate to, he clearly was the steadier of the two parents, a more positive role model. He spent many hours teaching Josh and David the history of the world, sharing his love of philosophy, religion and psychology. Josh felt a sadistic connection to his father, despite the dad's passivity in family interactions (he didn't intervene when the mother made decisions that were ineffective or hurtful.)

As an only child, his mother adored Josh, elevating him to the position of child-genius. *In many ways, he felt bonded to his mother in an unconscious marriage.* When David was born, he lost this status and David now received the attention that he had once enjoyed. She displayed the same dynamic as a grandmother to his children. He observed her drop attention from the firstborn after the second child was born. The oldest grandchild was devastated and became reactively depressed.

Josh remembered more and more examples of his mother aggravating the sibling rivalry. Dealing with David's gifted nature made it even more difficult for Josh to gain what he considered his *fair share* of maternal attention. Further complicating the neurosis, his mother demanded complete submission to her authority in the home. Any demonstration of unauthorized self-initiative was punished with cruelty. Josh's sense of self was quite damaged by this triangulation between his mother, David, and himself.

Josh was seething with unconscious hatred for David, who had supplanted him from the throne of his mother's excessive adoration. As therapy intensified, plot after plot emerged from the unconscious, focusing on David's death and his own restoration to pre-David glory. Mixed with this anger was profound survivor guilt. Josh unconsciously blamed himself for David's schizophrenia. He feared it was the result of his intense jealousy. He obsessed on other possibilities: his mother's seductive and volatile behavior, or his father's distant obsessive rigidity. Josh was truly tortured by feelings of guilt.

Josh married late in life, convinced that if he had not been pursued by his wife, he may never have married at all. Unfortunately, as time went on, he also became emotionally unavailable to his wife. He was again responding to feelings of sibling rivalry, *but now it was with his wife.* They would bicker endlessly over who was right and who was wrong in family disputes, what was fair and what was unfair. This interminable marital stalemate produced a twofold super-ego punishment: One, the destruction of closeness from his wife punished him for his fantasy of fratricide. (Remember Cain could not till fertile soil as punishment for the murder of Abel.) And two, the distance created by the bickering sustained his unconscious loyalty (incestuous attachment) to his mother. Obviously Josh could not be married to two women.

In therapy, Josh was able to mourn his father's death and overcome the rage he held in check for so long. He was now able to forgive himself for his jealous feelings toward his gifted, but severely impaired brother. He flew east to meet with his mother and explained face to face how much he loved his wife and family. He offered her a place in his life as *mother* and *grandmother* to the children. He stressed the importance of not hurting the relationship between his two children by lavishing attention on the youngest to the detriment of the oldest child.

He discovered that his mother was also a victim of a childhood trauma. Her father was an unstable individual who was unfaithful to his wife, a depressed woman. The pattern of favoring one child over another is replayed. With her older brother receiving the special attention, her emotional needs were unmet. Unconsciously, *her doting on David was a repair—showing how she had wanted to be treated by her parents.*

Josh no longer suffers from depression and has completed treatment successfully. His marriage is rich and intimate, and he is able to show his love to his wife and children with equal intensity. At work, he is respected by his fellow physicians.

Conclusion

There are many examples of how sibling conflicts become embedded in the unconscious life of neurotic individuals. It is essential to recognize that sibling induced trauma is a common, everyday reality that we all deal with in the human condition. It does not necessarily become part of a neurosis. I treat numerous patients who have warm and caring relationships with their siblings, many of whom were cruel to one another during their childhood. The competition, sadism, and meanness is balanced by companionship, playfulness and love. Sibling relationships teach social cooperation and teamwork in healthy family systems. Many times siblings balance out the deficiencies in either parent and can be life and *psyche-saving* for the child. It is true that sibling relationships are potential hotbeds of neurotic conflict. Sibling rivalry gets pulled into the vortex of a developing neurosis when the child is a participant in a triangle. The natural rivalry is aggravated because of the unconscious needs of one of the parents in the Oedipal phase.

The suffering that then ensues in the life of these patients can be devastating. The Biblical stories of Cain and Abel, Jacob and Esau, Joseph and his many brothers attest to the centrality of sibling rivalry to the human unconscious. It appears to be true that *we are our brother's keeper.* The super-ego would not have it any other way.

BIBLIOGRAPHY

Abend, S. (1984). Sibling love and object choice. *Psychoanal. Q.,* 53:425–430.

Adler, A. (1959). *Understanding Human Nature.* New York: Fawcett.

Agger, E. M. (1988). Psychoanalytic perspectives on sibling relationships. *Psychoanal. Inq.,* 8:3–30.

Bank, S. P. & Kahn, M. D. (1980–1981). Freudian siblings. *Psychoanal. Rev.,* 504. (1982). *The Sibling Bond.* New York: Basic Books.

Bernays, A. (1940). My brother, Sigmund Freud. *Amer. Mercury,* November, pp. 334–340.

Bieber, I. (1980). *Cognitive Psychoanalysis.* New York: Aronson.

Blos, P. (1979). *The Adolescent Passage.* New York, Int. Univ. Press.

Boer, F. & Dunne, J., Eds. (1992). *Children's Sibling Relationships.* Hillsdale, NJ: Erlbaum.

Bonaparte, M. (1953). *Female Sexuality.* New York: Int. Univ. Press.

Brazelton, T. B. (1969). *Infants and Mothers.* New York: Delta Books.

Buck, P. (1971). *The Story Bible, Volume I: The Old Testament.* New York: Signet Books.

Colarusso, C. & Nemiroff, C. (1981). *Adult Development.* New York: Plenum.

Colonna, A. B. & Newman, L. (1983). Psychoanalytic literature on siblings. *Psychoanal. Study Child,* 38:285–310.

Davanloo, H. (1990). *Unlocking the Unconscious.* Chichester, England. John Wiley & Sons.

Fenichel, O. (1931). Specific forms of the Oedipus complex. *Int. J. Psychoanal.,* 12:412–430.

Freud, S. (1915–1916). Introductory lectures on psycho-analysis. *S. E.,* 15.

——— (1935). An autobiographical study. *S. E.,* 15.

Frijling-Schreuder, E. C. M. (1972). The vicissitudes of aggression in normal development, in childhood neurosis and in childhood psychosis. *Int. J. Psychoanal.,* 53:185–190.

Graham, I. (1988). The sibling object and its transferences: alternate organizer of the middle field. *Psychoanal. Inq.,* 8:88–107.

Jacobson, E. (1964). *The Self and the Object World.* New York: Int. Univ. Press.

Jones, E. (1953). *The Life and Work of Sigmund Freud,* Vol. 1. New York: Basic Books.

Kernberg, O. F. (1976). *Object Relations Theory and Clinical Psychoanalysis.* New York: Aronson.

——— (1980). *Internal World and External Reality.* New York: Aronson.

Leichtman, M. (1985). Influence of an older sibling on the separation-individuation process. *Psychoanal. Study Child,* 40:111–162.

Loewald, H. W. (1979). The waning of the Oedipus complex. *J. Amer. Psychoanal. Assn.,* 27:751–776.

Mahler, M. S., Pine, F. & Bergman, A. (1975). *The Psychological Birth of the Human Infant.* New York: Basic Books.

Mallinger, A. C. (1978). Fear of success and oedipal experience. *J. Psychol.,* 100:91–106.

Neubauer, P. B. (1982). Rivalry, envy, and jealousy. *Psychoanal. Study Child,* 37:121–143.

——— (1983). The importance of the sibling experience. *Psychoanal. Study Child,* 38:325–336.

Parens, H. (1988). Siblings in early childhood: some direct observational findings. *Psychoanal. Inq.,* 8:31–50.

Ritvo, S. (1969). In A psychoanalytic view of the family: a study of family member interaction. *Psychoanal. Forum,* 3:11–65.

Rothstein, A. (1979). Oedipal conflicts in narcissistic personality disorders. *Int. J. Psychoanal.,* 60:189–200.

Schachter, F. F. (1982). Sibling de-identification and split-parent identification: a family tetrad. In *Sibling Relationships: Their Nature and Significance Across the Lifespan,* ed. M. E. Lamb & B. Sutton-Smith. Hillsdale, NJ, Erlbaum, pp. 123–152.

Sharpe, S & Rosenblatt, A. (1994). Oedipal Sibling Triangles. *J Amer Psychoanal Assn.* 42 (2): 491–523

Sharpless, E. (1990). The evolution of triadic object relations in the preoedipal phase: contributions of developmental research. *Psychoanal. Contemp. Thought,* 13:439–458.

Shopper, M. (1974). Twinning reaction in non twin siblings. *J. Amer. Acad. Child Psychiat.,* 13:300–318.

From *The Handbook of Infant Child and Adolescent Psychotherapy: Vol. 2,* ed. B. S. Mark, and J. A. Incorvaia, New York: Jason Aaronson, 1997. Reprinted with the publisher's permission.

Peri-natal Trauma, Anxiety and Resistance Against Emotional Closeness

The purpose of my presentation is to integrate attachment theory, affect theory, trauma theory, and neurobiology into an understandable therapeutic approach that offers effective short-term treatment to patients. I also want to explore the area of pre-verbal trauma beginning in the pre-natal phase of development and continuing into the first three months of life.

This patient presented to treatment with anxiety, hysteria, compulsive rescuing and marital maladjustment.

Modern Attachment Theory and the Concept of Trauma

Modern attachment theory focuses on the process of attunement, which is the largely nonverbal, right hemispheric mode of communication between caregiver and child (Schore, 1997). Affect regulation through psychic and somatic mechanisms is of critical importance in healthy development. When the child and his environment are out of balance, and *no repair takes place,* small t trauma occurs, resulting in anger and eventually defenses are formed. What leads to a traumatized state of mind? The key ingredient seems to be a state of helplessness in the face of actual (or imagined) danger (Freud, 1926). Anna Freud (1967) pointed out that "trauma" is used in two distinct ways by clinicians. In common usage it means an event that causes emotional disruption. Today we refer to this as small t trauma. The second usage is what we call big T trauma—an overwhelmed state wherein the individual is powerless to exert control over his environment.

Attunement failures between parent and child are always small t traumas. If they are repetitive, fixed, and rigid, there is no way to process the negative emotion that the trauma creates, and the effects become cumulative (Kahn, 1963). Ideally, small t and even large T traumatizing experiences are processed in the parent child dyad. However, when there is *impairment of parental empathy* these affects are not processed interpersonally, they are stored. In an attempt to define trauma in a non-trivial way, Joseph Jones (1995, p. 116) explains, "a traumatized state occurs when a person is unable to respond appropriately to a situation; in turn, this inability to respond is signaled by anxiety-panic." Depending upon 1) the child's temperament, 2) the degree of the trauma, and 3) the capacity of the caregivers to respond, an insecure attachment may form. I have coined the term "primitive aggressive self-organization (PASO)" to describe this acquired form of insecure attachment. I will have more to say about this term later in the paper. In the optimal parent child dyad, in Francine Shapiro's metaphor, the negative affects may be "digested" and no pathology results. Table 1 categorizes the types of traumas that patients bring with them to therapists in clinical practices.

I have chosen to present a patient whose core areas of trauma have had major pathogenic effects on the development of unregulated moods and an impaired capacity for intimate relatedness. This case illustrates core concepts of short-term therapy, as well as raising important questions. To reiterate, big T trauma refers to the kind of experiences in DSM IV that cause posttraumatic stress disorder: catastrophic experiences outside the realm of ordinary experience. Little t trauma is a result of those childhood events that produce a sense of helplessness, anxiety, shame, humiliation, and/ or abandonment, for which there has been no satisfactory repair from either parent. Much of this little t trauma is split off from consciousness and stored in largely inaccessible (non linguistic) form in the right hemisphere (Siegel, 1995, 1999). It is important to note that big T trauma inevitably activates dormant little t trauma.

It is my assertion that patients who are exposed to small t trauma (cumulative trauma, Kahn, 1963) have an insecure attachment underlying their mood and behavioral disorders. I believe that effective psycho-

Table 1. The Spectrum of Trauma: ***Conceptualization of Trauma: Little "t" progressing to Big "T"***

Relating
Faulty attunement by either or both caregivers
Faulty empathy by either or both caregivers
Parenting
Faulty application of boundaries from caregivers
Favoritism; sibling rivalry
Defective affect regulation
Exploitative
Sexual abuse
Physical abuse
Power: Children as pawns or scapegoats
Triangulation
Environmental
Death of parent or sibling
Injury of person or body part
Divorce
Poverty
Natural disasters
Social discrimination: sex, race, culture

therapeutic treatment can only occur when the patient faces the complex feelings that are "inside the insecure attachment." The resolution of successful psychotherapy means that the patient and therapist have created an "earned secure attachment" (Pearson, 1994). The secure attachment phenomenon is undoubtedly mediated by the neurotransmitters in the limbic system, and primarily serotonin, norepinephrine, and dopamine.[1] Much of psychopharmacology actually manipulates this system.

1. Acetylcholine is an important cortical neurotransmitter involved with affect regulation as well. It may mediate major defensive operation as well as shame, guilt and despair (Neborsky and Janowsky, 1980).

Serotonin reuptake inhibitors ameliorate anxiety, decrease aggression and induce secure attachment phenomenon. Although in theory this is a wonderful thing, the effect is largely "state dependent" and new learning often doesn't take place and unfortunately the patient remains dependent on the drug for freedom from depression and anxiety.

On the other hand, many psychotherapies with these patients fail as well because the therapists either lack the technical or theoretical skill to overcome the patient's resistance to experiencing the feelings that exist inside the unconscious insecure attachment. Many therapies do not address resistance-or purport to address resistance-but in fact do not overcome the barrier to genuine feeling. I frequently see patients who have had years of psychoanalysis and the core attachment pathology has not yielded to psychoanalytic technique.

In the book, *Short-Term Therapy for Long-Term Change,* I introduce the term "PASO" as a short hand for the complex mixture of feelings and defenses that exist inside the insecure attachment. It is important to emphasize that these feelings are not conscious. They are highly conflicted and are either repressed or dissociated. It is my belief that all successful therapies restore the patient to a state of secure attachment, and restore their ability to experience contentment, to have joyful intimate relationships, to exert healthy self-assertion increases and they become resilient to stress-laden situations.

Habib Davanloo (1995) first described the "PASO"—without actually using the term—in his pioneering efforts to develop a short-term psychotherapy. Clinicians like myself who trained with Davanloo have developed our own spin-off therapies that rely on his original discoveries.

The foundation of short-term dynamic psychotherapy therapy lies in the belief that the patient must experience their *genuine feelings from the past, in the present.* My video demonstration of an initial interview with a patient with severe anxiety, hysteria and compulsive rescuing will show how this is accomplished. In my work, I have added an important component to the goal of *genuine feelings from the past, in the present*: I want the patient to leave their "initial interview" with a coherent narrative of the origin of his or her psychopathology. A coherent narrative is an understanding of the origins of their difficulties that includes the unconscious perspective. The patient will understand the dynamic origin of their anxiety, they will understand the role of either guilt or shame in their depression or self abuse. The patient will understand what drives their compulsions. The patient will understand unconscious anger and its relationship to their other affects.

These insights and understandings will be experiential as opposed to intellectual. In some cases (but not all) the transgenerational transmission of the trauma will become clear. All comprehensive treatments will eventually trace the origin of their difficulties back to the grandparents. In fact, patients successfully receiving this treatment are freed from the unconscious transmission of the trauma to their children. Currently I am working on a series of cases where I have video-recorded the actual "unlocking of the unconscious[2]" of parents and their adult neurotic children (Lifespan Learning Institute: Hysteria Conference, Los Angeles, October 2000), and the transgenerational transmission of unconscious trauma is startlingly apparent.

Now let's take a closer look at the PASO and see how it operates and then I will present how I believe little t trauma is transferred from one generation to the next.

I want to thank Marion Solomon (co-author of *Short-Term Therapy for Long-Term Change*) for her illustration of the PASO and the idea of using Russian dolls. Let's examine the PASO in more detail.

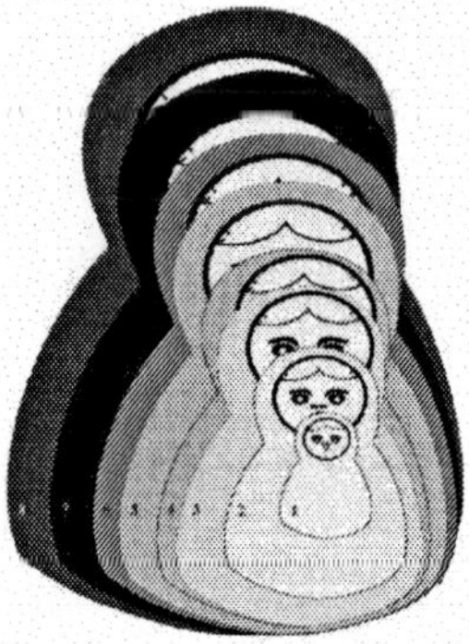

Figure 1. The "PASO"

2. A term invented by Davanloo (1995) to describe the process that I will present in the video.

1. At the center of the PASO (insecure attachment) lies *the capacity for secure attachment.* When this is present, the individual has the capacity for contentment. Relationships are intimate and empathy for the feeling processes of others is intact.
2. Next lies the emotion of *pain.* Classically, pain is not considered an emotion against which people defend, but in our system it is. We record the emotion of pain, and call it the "pain of trauma."
3. Closely allied to pain is *sadness.* This sadness is the result of loss of the closeness with the attachment figure.
4. The *retaliatory rage* that is repressed in the unconscious can be found at this level. The rage is frequently left unnoticed in traditional therapy. In Bowlby's (1973) model, the unprocessed existence of this rage for an extended period of time leads to despair.
5. *Anxiety* is found at this ring of the PASO that surrounds the sadness and/or the rage.
6. This level contains the *"crippling inhibitory affects"* of shame or guilt.
7. Overlaying the aforementioned affects are the defenses. There are several layers of *defenses: the tactical, the dynamic and the characterologic.*
8. Layer eight is seen only in more highly resistant cases: we call this the *defense against emotional closeness.* It is a defensive position in which detachment from all relatedness pervades the person's psyche.

Although not schematized, grief is also frequently encountered between the defenses and the guilt-shame layer. This sadness is a function of the lost time and opportunity the patient has suffered from the existence of their defenses. Sexual feeling is located between layers four and five. Sexuality and aggressive feeling can be commingled when certain types of abuse and empathic failures occur.

Short-term dynamic psychotherapy explores this structure in each and every psychotherapy session. The way this is done varies with different styles of short-term therapy. But all short-term therapies focus on the patient's resistance (defenses) and techniques are used to overcome those defenses. It is the defenses that interfere with the patient's ability to process painful affects and restore a healthy operative self. The technique of e-stdp allows dissociated and repressed affects to become conscious and to be "re-processed." Short-term dynamic psychotherapy operates in much the same way. The cure is promoted by the patient's ability to access the emotions described in the PASO—layers 1 through 6.

I want to focus on two particular aspects of the unconscious for the purposes of this conference. One is the pre-natal and post-natal experience of multiple big T traumas, and the other is the transmission of hysteria from mother to child.

Mary Main (1991, 1993, in press) has discussed data that shows that psychopathology can be predicted in children of mothers with an incoherent narrative. The incoherent narrative is thought to reflect unresolved trauma in the mother. Mothers with unresolved trauma defend against the affects that are mobilized in that area of trauma. However the trauma that is not processed is repeated in behavior. The mothers, in effect, treat their children the same way they had been treated themselves. However, there is little in the literature, which supports peri-natal and pre-natal trauma as etiologic in psychoneurosis.

Otto Rank (1924) challenged Freud with his emphasis on birth trauma as the core of neurosis rather than sexual trauma. These ideas have not held much of a following. Newer neuroscience research (Schore, oral communication) supports the idea that the right hemisphere of the brain in third trimester is mature enough to encode olfactory and sensory memory. In studies related to adoption, it seems attachment is less specific before the fourth month of life. It seems that prior to four months the neurological organization of the infant's brain does not make a specific code of the mother's face. This means that transfer of the infant is less disruptive before four months. However, auditory awareness, olfactory awareness, and somatosensory awareness are operating and recording sensory impressions.

History: Big T Trauma

Her mother first abandoned the patient in this presentation soon after birth. The mother (and father) left their neo-natal twins in the hospital and returned to their home in another country to get emergency surgery. One twin died hours after birth and the other—the patient—was believed to be too frail to live. After the mother left, a stewardess from their airline heard the story and came to the hospital daily to bond with the child. The patient survived and thrived. The first separation trauma, then, was from her twin at birth, and the second occurred when she was parted from her surrogate mother, who was calm and protective, to be reunited with her birth mother at three months of age.

It must have been a difficult transition for her from the secure attachment with her calm Good Samaritan mother to her high strung, temperamental and controlling biological mother. Further compounding the problem in this particular case, the patient felt responsible (reinforcement of unconscious omnipotence) for the death of her identical twin sister who died a few hours after birth. Remarkably, in the unlocking of her unconscious, the implicit memory of that sibling returns and the patient also recovers implicit memory of the Good Samaritan mother who adopted her in the intensive care nursery and bonded with her in the first weeks of her life. Did this patient bond on that level to her Good Samaritan mother? Was the separation a big T trauma? Can ISTDP access and repair trauma from three months of life?

History: Little t (Relational) Trauma

Her mother is described by the patient as an immature narcissistic woman with hypochondrical and histrionic features. She controlled the child with her emotionalism. This mal-attunement created anger without repair and thus increased in intensity and power. The intensity of the anger became associated with death wishes toward the mother. The mother's hypochondriasis compounded the fear (anxiety) over the death wishes (insecure attachment, avoidant type). The patient loved her mother and began to feel guilty over her angry feelings toward her. Unconsciously this guilt resonated with the unconscious "murder" of her sister. Next the mother and daughter became embroiled in a power struggle over playing the violin. (This probably represents a re-enactment of a power struggle with mother's mother.) The patient reports a time when her mother forced her to practice her violin despite having an acutely broken arm. The patient developed negative oppositional autonomy. She stubbornly refused to conform to her mother's wishes and became overtly rebellious. The patient's father was the steadier of the two parents, but he was passive and never advocated for the patient during a conflict.

Over time, the patient naturally begins to grow, develop, separate, and individuate. However, the damage was already done (Sroufe, 1990). Her self-regulatory processes are disordered. She too had developed hysterical characteristics, prone to tantrums and emotional outbursts. Another way of thinking about this issue is that she has failed to separate and individuate in a positive frame. Instead, she is always with the mother who controlled and manipulated her, and she is full of unconscious anger directed now not outwardly against mother, but against herself. The guilt over the rage against mother is continuously undone by attempts at rescuing others who are like her. Prior to therapy, she was attracted to abusive and neglectful love relationships. Her first marriage was to a gay male. She believed she could help him become better adjusted. He abruptly left (abandonment) her alone in a strange country (re-enactment). Not long after she got on her feet, she fell in love and became pregnant by a man whose developmental history closely mirrored hers. Their relationship was for the first time in his life one which broke through his resistance to emotional closeness. At first there was deep passion and intimacy. But after they married and the child was born, severe triangulation between the husband and his parents occurred, and the patient again experienced distance, isolation, and aloneness, which recapitulated her earlier abandonments.

On a deeper level, her husband initially was the Good Samaritan mother, but over time he became the birth mother who abandoned her in the ICU (mother of neglect). She came to treatment after her husband completed a course of ISTDP with me in which he successfully addressed his core unconscious issues.

What, one might ask, drives this unconscious process over years and years, and why doesn't the patient just learn new behaviors? The answer is, she can't. First, the information she needs to unlearn is split-off into non-verbal right hemisphere memory. Second, the pathology is maintained by the propensity for transference, projection and projective identification with caregivers and authority figures in her life. There is a powerful unconscious force in trauma patients called *narrative re-enactment.* Freud (1918) recognized it, as did Erik Erikson (1963) as did Davanloo (Oral communication). So the patient is driven to attach herself to figures that resemble her mother and sister so she can re-enact the original trauma. The reasons behind this are controversial. Davanloo believes that the compulsion to repeat is a superego phenomenon to punish the self over and over again for the unconscious anger at the offending relative. Earlier theorists like Freud (1911, 1926) and Erikson (1963) saw it as an attempt to master the trauma. It is probably a combination of both, particularly in patients who present for therapy.

The compulsive behavior (rescuing) serves another function as well. Since there is no internal, stable secure attachment the patient has to rely on external sources for stability. Her feelings themselves are not a secure place. Compulsion is predictable, stable and reliable. Therefore the compulsive behavior compensates for the missing capacity to support and sooth oneself in the face of adversity, keeps distance from others, and undoes the unconscious guilt over the destruction of her sister and fantasized destruction of caregivers. The hysteria is also a reflection of impaired capacity to sooth oneself and reflectively considers one's options. The hysteria is a negative identification with her mother who controlled everyone in her family with her emotionalism. But the underlying core of the psychopathology seems to be grief and guilt over the loss of her twin.

The videotape, which follows the slide presentation, is a forty-five-minute synopsis of a six-hour trial therapy of a thirty-year-old female referred for intensive short-term dynamic psychotherapy. It is edited to show exposure of the PASO and the emotional insight into the peri-natal origin of her problems. I hope you find the videotape interesting and moving. A six-month follow up vignette will be shown.

BIBLIOGRAPHY

Ainsworth, M. D. S., Blehar, M. C., Waters, E., & Wall, S. (1978). *Patterns of attachment: A psychological study of the Strange Situation.* Hillsdale, NJ: Erlbaum.

Ainsworth, M. D. S. & Eichberg, C. (1991). Effects on infant-mother attachment of mother's unresolved loss of an attachment figure, or other traumatic experience. In C. M. Parkes, J. Stevenson-Hinde, & P. Marris (Eds.), *Attachment across the life cycle* (pp. 160–186). London: Routledge.

Bowlby, J. (1969). *Attachment and loss: Vol. 1. Attachment.* New York: Basic Books.

Bowlby, J. (1973). *Attachment and loss: Vol. 2. Separation and anger.* New York: Basic Books.

Bowlby, J. (1980). *Attachment and loss: Vol. 3. Loss: Sadness and depression.* New York: Basic Books.

Bowlby, J. (1988). *A secure base: Parent-child attachment and healthy human development.* New York: Basic Books.

Davanloo, H. (1988a). Clinical manifestations of superego pathology. Part II. The resistance of the superego and the liberation of the paralyzed ego. *International Journal of Short-Term Psychotherapy, 3,* 1–24.

Davanloo, H. (1988b). The technique of unlocking the unconscious. Part II. Partial unlocking of the unconscious. *International Journal of Short-Term Psychotherapy, 3 (2),* 123–159.

Davanloo, H. (1988b). The technique of unlocking of the unconscious. Part I. *International Journal of Short-Term Psychotherapy, 3 (2),* 99–121.

Davanloo, H. (1988c). The technique of unlocking of the unconscious. Part II. Partial unlocking of the unconscious. *International Journal of Short-Term Psychotherapy, 3 (2),* 123–159.

Davanloo, H. (1989a). Central dynamic sequence in the unlocking of the unconscious and comprehensive trial therapy. Part I. Major unlocking. *International Journal of Short-Term Psychotherapy, 4 (1),* 1–33.

Davanloo, H. (1989b). Central dynamic sequence in the major unlocking of the unconscious and comprehensive trial therapy. Part II. The course of trial therapy after the initial breakthrough. *International Journal of Short-Term Psychotherapy, 4 (1),* 35–66.

Davanloo, H. (1989c). The technique of unlocking the unconscious in patients suffering from functional disorder. Part I. Restructuring ego's defenses. *International Journal of Short-Term Psychotherapy, 4 (2),* 93–116.

Davanloo, H. (1989d). The technique of unlocking the unconscious in patients suffering from functional disorders. Part II. Direct view of the dynamic unconscious. *International Journal of Short-Term Psychotherapy, 4 (2),* 117–148.

Davanloo, H. (1990). *Unlocking the Unconscious.* Chichester: Wiley.

Davanloo, H. (1995a). Intensive short-term dynamic psychotherapy: spectrum of psycho-neurotic disorders. *International Journal of Short-Term Psychotherapy, 10 (3, 4),* 121–155.

Davanloo, H. (1995b). Intensive short-term dynamic psychotherapy: technique of partial and major unlocking of the unconscious with a highly resistant patient. Part I. Partial unlocking of the unconscious. *International Journal of Short-Term Psychotherapy, 10 (3, 4),* 157–181.

Davanloo, H. (1995c). Intensive short-term dynamic psychotherapy: major unlocking of the unconscious. Part II. The course of the trial therapy after partial unlocking. *International Journal of Short-Term Psychotherapy, 10 (3, 4),* 183–230.

Davanloo, H. (1996a). Management of tactical defenses in intensive short-term dynamic psychotherapy. Part I. Overview, tactical defenses of cover words and indirect speech. *International Journal of Short-Term Psychotherapy, 11 (3),* 129–152.

Davanloo, H. (1996b). Management of tactical defenses in intensive short-term dynamic psychotherapy. Part II. Spectrum of tactical defenses. *International Journal of Short-Term Psychotherapy, 11 (3),* 153–199.

Davanloo, H. (1999). Intensive short-term dynamic psychotherapy—central dynamic sequence: Phase of pressure. *International Journal of Short-Term Psychotherapy, 13:4,* 211–233.

Davanloo, H. (1999). Intensive short-term dynamic psychotherapy—central dynamic sequence: Phase of challenge. *International Journal of Short-Term Psychotherapy, 13:4,* 237–260.

Davanloo, H. (1999). Intensive short-term dynamic psychotherapy—central dynamic sequence: Head-on collision with resistance. *International Journal of Short-Term Psychotherapy, 13:4,* 263–280.

Emde, R. (1983). The prerepresentational self and its affective core. *The Psychoanalytic Study of the Child,* 38:165–192. New haven, CT: Yale University Press.

Erikson, E. H. (1963). *Childhood and society.* 2nd ed. New York: W. W. Norton & Company.

Freud, A. (1967). Comment on trauma. In: *Psychic Trauma,* ed. S.S. Furst. New York: Basic Books, pp. 235–245.0

Freud, S. (1911). *Remembering, Repeating, and Working Through. Standard Edition,* 12:150. London: Hogarth Press, 1959.

Freud, S. (1918). *Introduction to Psychoanalysis and the War Neurosis. Standard Edition,* 17:207–210. London: Hogarth Press, 1959.

Freud, S. (1926). *Inhibitions, Symptoms, and Anxiety. Standard Edition,* 20:75–175. London: Hogarth Press, 1959.

Janowsky, D., and Neborsky, R.J., (1980) Hypothesized common mechanisms in the psychopharmacologic and psychotherapeutic treatment of depression. *Psychiatric Annals, 10:9356–361.*

Jones, J.M. (1995). *Affects as process.* Hillsdale, New Jersey: Analytic Press.

Kahn, M (1963). The concept of cumulative trauma. *The Psychoanalytic Study of the Child,*. New haven, CT: Yale University Press.

Main, M. (1991). Metacognitive knowledge, metacognitive monitoring, and singular (coherent) versus multiple (incoherent) models of attachment: Findings and directions for future research. In C. M. Parkes, J. Stenson-Hinde, & P. Marris (Eds.), *Attachment across the life cycle* (pp. 127–159). London: Routledge.

Main, M. (1993). Discourse, prediction, and recent studies in attachment: Implications for psychoanalysis. *Journal of the American Psychoanalytic Association, 41,* 209–244.

Main, M. (1995). Attachment: Overview, with implications for clinical work. In S. Goldberg, R. Muir, & J. Kerr (Eds.), *Attachment theory: Social, developmental and clinical perspectives* (pp. 407–474). Hillsdale, NJ: Analytic Press.

Main, M. (1996). Introduction to the special section on attachment and psychopathology: 2. Overview of the field of attachment. *Journal of Consulting and Clinical Psychology, 64,* 237–243.

Main, M. (in press). The Adult Attachment Interview: Fear, attention, safety and discourse processes. *Journal of the American Psychoanalytic Association.*

Main, M. & Goldwyn, R. (1984). *Adult attachment scoring and classification system.* Unpublished manuscript, University of California at Berkeley.

Main, M. & Goldwyn, R. (1998). *Adult attachment scoring and classification systems* (Version 6.3). Unpublished manuscript, University of California at Berkeley.

Main, M. & Hesse, E. (1990). Parent's unresolved traumatic experiences are related to infant disorganized status: Is frightened and/or frightening parental behavior the linking mechanism? In M. T. Greenberg, D. Cicchetti, & E. M. Cummings (Eds.), *Attachment in the preschool years: Theory, research, and intervention* (pp. 161–182). Chicago: University of Chicago Press.

Main, M., Kaplan, N., & Cassidy, J. (1985). Security in infancy, childhood, and adulthood: A move to the level of representation. In I. Bretherton & E. Waters (Eds.), Growing points of attachment theory and research. *Monographs of the Society for Research in Child Development, 50* (2–3 Serial No. 209), 66–104.

Main, M. & Morgan, H. (1996). Disorganization and disorientation in infant Strange Situation behavior: Phenotypic resemblance to dissociative states. In L. K. Michelson & W. J. Ray (Eds.), *Handbook of dissociation: Theoretical, empirical, and clinical perspectives* (pp. 121–160). Chicago: University of Chicago Press.

Main, M. & Solomon, J. (1986). Discovery of an insecure-disorganized/disoriented attachment pattern. In T. B. Brazelton & M. Yogman (Eds.), *Affective development in infancy* (pp. 95–124). Norwood, NJ: Ablex.

Main, M. & Solomon, J. (1990). Procedures for identifying infants as disorganized/disoriented during the Ainsworth Strange Situation. In M. T. Greenberg, D. Cicchetti, & E. M. Cummings (Eds.), *Attachment in the preschool years: Theory, research, and intervention* (pp. 121–160). Chicago: University of Chicago Press.

Neborsky, R.J., (1982) *Hypothesized common mechanisms in the psychopharmacologic and psychotherapeutic treatment of depression.* Grand Rounds, George Washington School of Medicine.

Neborsky, R.J. (1998) A new metapsychology of the unconscious. UCSD Cutting Edge Conference. *Short-Term Therapy for Long-Term Change.* La Jolla, California.

Neborsky, R.J. (2000) A study in hysteria. One-day symposium. Lifespan Learning Institute. November 2, Los Angeles, California.

Pearson, J.L., Cohn, D.A., Cowan, P.A., & Cowan, C. P. (1994). Earned and continuous security in adult attachment: Relation to depressive symptomotology and parenting style. *Development and Psychopathology,* 6, 259–373.

Rank, O. (1924) *The trauma of birth.* New York: Robert Brunner.

Schore, A. N. (1996). The experience-dependent maturation of a regulatory system in the orbital prefrontal cortex and the origin of developmental psychopathology. *Development and Psychopathology, 8,* 59–87.

Schore, A. N. (1997). Early organization of the nonlinear right brain and development of a predisposition to psychiatric disorders. *Development and Psychopathology, 9,* 595–631.

Schore, A. N. (1998). The experience-dependent maturation of an evaluative system in the cortex. In K. H. Pribram & J. King (Eds.), *Brain and values: Is a biological science of values possible?* (pp. 337–358). Mahway, NJ: Erlbaum.

Schore, A. N. (in press). Clinical Implications of a neurobiological model of projective identification. In S. Alhanti, Ed *Primitive Mental States,*

Volume III "Pre- and Peri-natal influences on personality development." ESF Publishers.

Shapiro, F. (1995) *Eye Movement Desensitization and Reprocessing: Basic Principles, Protocols and Procedures.* New York: Guilford.

Siegel, D. J. (1995). Memory, trauma, and psychotherapy: A cognitive science view. *Journal of Psychotherapy Practice and Research, 4,* 93–122.

Siegel, D. J. (1999). *The developing mind.* New York: Guilford Press.

Solomon, M.F., Neborsky, R. J., McCullough, L., Alpert, M., Shapiro, F., Malan, D.M., (2001 in press) *Short-Term Therapy for Long-Term Change.* New York: W.W. Norton and Co.

Stern, D. N. (1985). *The interpersonal world of the infant.* New York: Basic Books.

Sroufe, L.A., Egeland, B., & Krentger, T. (1990). The fate of early experience following developmental change: Longitudinal approaches to individual adaptation in childhood. *Child Development,* 54, 1615–1627.

From *Core Factors for Effective Short-Term Dynamic Psychotherapy.* Quaderni di Psichiatria Pratica, Vl n. 17/18, pp. 80–96. December 2001.

Healing Trauma

A Clinical Model for the Comprehensive Treatment of Trauma Using an Affect-Experiencing Attachment Theory Approach

In this troubled period, post-September 11, 2001, this chapter is particularly timely. On that day all of us were exposed in one way or another to the devastating effects of what Francine Shapiro refers to as "big T trauma." A large percentage of the nation's population suffered from the signs and symptoms of acute trauma exposure. These symptoms are well-known to us and they include anxiety, lowered mood, obsessive thoughts, anger, grief, flashbacks of the events, sleep disorders and nightmares. As time went on many of us resolved these symptoms. However, a small percentage of people developed clinical anxiety disorders (PTSD) or depression, and required professional intervention.

Who make up this small percentage? In his longitudinal studies of trauma-exposed individuals, Martin Korn, MD (2001) states that one factor stands out in the prediction of who will develop pathology post trauma exposure—neuroticism. He defines this trait as measured on different personality scales as the "tendency to experience negative affects when exposed to a new event." Apparently this trait is stable across the lifespan from infancy to senescence. It is a very powerful predictor and in fact accounts for twice the variance as the actual stressor accounts for. This epidemiological research finding is consistent with clinical observation and attachment research. It is my hope to offer a new approach to the comprehensive treatment of trauma victims that includes intervention at the level of *neuroticism.* It is my central thesis that within each of us there is an unconscious negative affect processing system that protects us from developing anxiety and/or depression. That system that is responsible for this function is called the attachment system. What must a healthy attachment system do when exposed to trauma in order to preserve mental health[1].

1) All of the negative emotion that the event created *and activated* must be "metabolized."[2]
2) The event must be framed in a way that is consistent with the patients' core belief system. Their core belief system is the working model of how the world works. This exists on a continuum from the random universe theory to a perfect order theory (a higher power decides what happens). Their psychologic process must address and formulate beliefs about: A) where the focus of control resides; B) the sources of danger and what exposure to danger means; and C) the meaning of life.

In this chapter I will demonstrate why I believe both of those tasks are a function of a healthy, integrated attachment system. By way of a preview, I will first outline how trauma is processed with an integrated attachment system. Next I will examine how and why chronic disorders of stress happen. And finally, I will address effective treatment vis-a-vis technique and illustrative clinical case examples.

1. A Model for Understanding the Effects of Trauma on Our Brains and Minds

Acute trauma by definition exposes the individual to an extraordinary event wherein their sense of control is violated. When that occurs there is a discharge of extreme intense emotion: grief, anger, or fear. This then activates latent unconscious mechanisms for self-repair which, since the

---

1. I am using Dan Siegel's functional definition of mental health as "adaptability, flexibility and stability of the nervous system over time."

2. Closely related to Francine Shapiro's concept that negative affects must be "digested."

time of Freud, have been called defense mechanisms. The purpose of defense mechanisms is to restore homeostasis as soon as possible to preserve adaptive capacity. Allan Schore has outlined the stress response circuitry of the infant showing how essential it is for the child to decrease arousal to preserve neural growth. This innate mechanism for self-preservation exists in trauma. A person is trapped in a burning building. Everything indicates he is going to die a horrible death. There is no escape. Arousal is off the scales, fear is pumping and suddenly a remarkable calm takes over. The person is calm, time seems to slow down, there is no pain and a comforting acceptance of his fate occurs.[3] In this hypothetical example, the mechanisms of dissociation and emotional detachment have intervened and prevented panic. If the person is miraculously saved, he will receive care and begin to go about his life. He will talk about his near miss, have dreams about fire, dreams about being trapped and rescued, and will process that event subconsciously until all the implicit memory of the event is detoxified. He will seek and find comfort in his relationships and support institutions that may or may not include counseling. After six months the emotion associated with the event is largely gone—fires in fireplaces do not trigger arousal or flashbacks, and the person has explained to himself why the event occurred and why he survived along the aforementioned philosophical continuums.

Now let's take that same person and imagine he was abused as a toddler—let's say age two to three—he was held down by his caregiver and punished for misbehavior with burning cigarettes. He dealt with the abuse the best he could, but suffers from mild anxiety, depression and negative thinking. The memory is so painful that he has blocked it and all negative emotions related to the event from consciousness. In the acute situation, the person's response to the fire is the same. After the rescue he begins to suffer from panic attacks that stop his functioning. Not only does he have bad dreams, but also horrible nightmares with torture and butchery. He is flooded with self-destructive impulses and may even attempt suicide. Finally, he seeks professional help and requires medications and extensive psychotherapy. Why? The acute traumatic event unlocked a hidden file in his implicit memory system for which there is no language, only image and feeling.

---

3. Probably mediated by discharge of endogenous opiates

Understanding this process is crucial to successful work with trauma victims so let me restate it clearly. The emotions associated with childhood trauma (relational failure, abuse or neglect) are either repressed or dissociated in an unconscious file. Two things can access and activate the negative emotional consequences of this hidden file: 1) experience of adult trauma, or 2) most importantly and surprisingly, by an intimate relationship. I will discuss this second activating dynamic later in this chapter.

When the file is activated by adult trauma, it is like a dam breaking (or Pandora's infamous box) and the affects can create anxiety, depression, somatic conversion symptoms, psycho physiologic disorder and/or self-abuse. With relational activation, it's more like a slow leak in which paradigms of abuse and neglect enter the person's life, and psychiatric symptoms appear as well. Unlike the first hypothetical person who was in the fire, this person's attachment system is overwhelmed by the unconscious affects stimulated by the trauma and a disorder of stress develops. A further complication of unresolved trauma is narrative re-enactment of the trauma wherein the victim unconsciously re-creates the traumatic event over and over again. Literally, they can jump from the frying pan into the fire and back again (Erikson, Davanloo, Vander, Kolk).

Table 1. The Two Responses to Acute Trauma of "Secures" versus "Insecures"

No Traumatic Attachment in Unconscious	*Traumatic Attachment in Unconscious*
Overwhelming Emotion	Overwhelming Emotion
No hidden files to activate	Activation of Hidden Files of Emotion
Temporary Defense	Temporary and Permanent Defense
Residual Anxiety, Disorder of Stress	Chronic Anxiety, Disorder of Stress
Stress Processing (Attachment System Intact)	Defective Stress Processing (Insecure)
Cognitive Reframing of Event	Unsuccessful Reframing
Return to Normal Baseline in 6 Months	No Return to Pre-morbid Baseline

2. A Model for Healing from Trauma

Attachment relationship information is recorded in an unconscious state, which is stored in implicit memory. It is, in effect, our stress-processing mechanism. Securely attached people metabolize life stresses well; insecurely attached individuals metabolize them less efficiently. Life difficulties and intimate relational conflicts mobilize the unconscious attachment system, and symptoms and narrative re-enactments occur. Ultimately, the more severe attachment disruptions lead to the kinds of neuropsychological deficits described by Fonagy, et al (2001). Because the attachment system is not "localized," but exists as parts of all aspects of emotional experience as reflected in mind-body states, the effects of attachment are *always* present in both gross and subtle ways.

This thesis is central to this chapter as well as to my research goal, which is to establish a comprehensive psychotherapy that alters malfunctioning attachment relationships. So let me outline here what I think happens normally to help trauma victims recover, and then what psychotherapy must do in order to facilitate that process. Our brains have in them inherent trauma processing systems. These are a function of secure attachment. If a child is disturbed by an environmental event, he or she returns to the attachment figure for comfort. Comfort takes many forms both overt and covert. On the overt level, mothers pick up their children, hold them, distract them, etc. On covert levels, processes like mirroring affect or containment behavior with vocal and tonal synchronization, are elicited until the child is restored to calmness and play or exploratory behavior resumes. It is clear (Main, 1985) that this process becomes internalized and becomes autonomous (*i.e.*, operates without mother or father present) and works at both a conscious and unconscious level. Intimately involved with stress-trauma management on a day-to-day basis are our biorhythms. Our REM[4] sleep in 90-minute burst, in a twenty-four hour cycle "digests" trauma that is experienced on a daily basis. In dreaming, the brain compares the trauma with early memory traces of similar experience, and files the memories of the day's events according to an affect-based associative system for further use and potential survival value. Comforting figures may appear in

---

4. In REM sleep information passes bi-hemispherically from the right hemisphere to the left and then back again. Perhaps, this is how EMDR helps with adaptive information processing.

the dream to give care, advice, counsel, and relief, if necessary. The nightly dream process helps the dreamer receive positive resolution of his or her experience, and they move on to the next day's activities restored, refreshed, and prepared for survival-based action.

The insecurely attached dreamer may or may not receive comfort for the day's stresses since the caregiver may have been the source of early stress or threat. It is highly likely that the dream will not achieve successful resolution, and hidden files (dissociated or repressed memories and affects) will be activated. The insecurely attached person must constantly recruit other sources of comfort within and/or outside of self for comfort. These are in the form of defenses or addictions. (See table 2). The person's impaired capacity to metabolize stress will eventually lead to instability, an inability to adapt, or some form of rigid, fixed response pattern. Illness of one kind or another results from defective core unconscious attachments.

Table 2. Cascade of Possible Maladaptive Defenses Following Trauma

Cognition	*Affective*	*Behavioral*
Intellectualization	Dissociation	Avoidance and Withdrawal
Rationalization	Introjection	Regression
Isolation of Affect	Projection	Isolation of Self
Attention Deficit	Somatization	Compulsion[5]
Denial	Detachment	Dependency
Isolation of Affect	Splitting	Impulsivity
Repression		Passivity
Vagueness		

I will now present two illustrative cases of insecure attachment, one with mixed therapeutic results, and the other with complete symptom removal and characterologic change following acute trauma. Both patients had a cold, controlling, and dismissive mothers. In the first case, the pa-

5. This includes all possible addictive strategies: alcohol, drugs, love, sex, eating disorders, work, religion, and even psychotherapy. See later discussion on the self-regulatory function of compulsion.

tient's father died when the patient was two years old, in the second case, the patient's father died when the patient was forty years old.

Clinical history 1: Insecure Attachment: Poorly Resolved Big T Trauma, Partial Treatment Response—Mixed Outcome.

Carol was a beautiful blonde blue-eyed teenager. Undoubtedly, she could have been a professional model. I saw her at age fifteen on an emergency evaluation. Her mother told me that she was found wandering the streets of our village in a disoriented state. Six months earlier she had been brutally gang raped by a wandering band of migrant workers who had illegally crossed the border from Mexico. She had been seeing a psychologist twice each week and had been rapidly deteriorating. She had begun drinking and abusing marijuana, but her evaluation showed primarily a dissociative fugue state. I hospitalized her and treated her as an in-patient. While Carol was in the hospital, I discovered that her biologic father died of a melanoma of the eye when she was nearly three. In all in-patient treatment modalities, she adamantly refused to discuss the rape. Upon discharge, Carol had reintegrated from her psychosis to a narcissistic personality. She was haughty, arrogant, dismissive and drove everyone, peer or adult, away from being close to her. She continued to be highly anxious and showed school problems, truancy, and many phobias. She bonded with a nice, but very passive underachieving boyfriend, and moved out of her home and in with him and his family. One day during outpatient therapy, she revealed the awful things that had happened to her. She cried, but the full ranges of emotions were never explored. Soon thereafter she stopped seeing me. A few years later she called me in an emergency. She was terrified. She had been working as a barmaid and told me the following story.

She went to Las Vegas with a man and married him on an impulse. It turned out that not only was he Mexican, but also a member of the Mexican Mafia and was wanted by multiple law enforcement agencies as a violent offender. She had tried to leave him but he threatened to kill her. Eventually she left him and was under police protection. A few days earlier, he had come to her house, kidnapped her, and taken her to the woods (near the original rape), tied her up and sodomized her. She now was under extreme police protection—a witness protection program—and was going to testify against him and have him brought to justice. A detective took a liking to her and acted as a father figure, looking after her. Nevertheless, she was flooded with panic symptoms as well as flashbacks of her original rape. Finally, she dealt with the terror, shame, and self-loathing from years ago. She returned to therapy and this time resolved the trauma, focusing on the loss of her father at age three, including her irrational guilt and self-blame over his death. Her perpetrator received life imprisonment. After this incident, she left the local area and became a flight attendant, met a supportive, loving Eastern European immigrant contractor and married. On follow up two years later, she returned with no obvious psychiatric problems, but was on complete medical disability for a neurological disorder of unclear origin. She was taking heavy doses of painkillers. Conversion disorder, malingering or addictive disease could not be ruled out.

Clinical History 2. Insecure Attachment, Completely Resolved Big T and Small t Trauma.

Cheryl, a therapist, had seen me for intensive short-term therapy to resolve problems with intimacy. It seems she had married two men who had little or no capacity for intimacy. Both marriages ended in divorce. We worked through underlying dynamics surrounding her anger at a cold, controlling and self-centered mother and anger at her father for his dependency and inability to stand up to his wife. The therapy seemed successful and Cheryl terminated. Two years later she called for an emergency appointment. She was suffering from acute PTSD. On the first visit she told me what had happened. Her father, a successful businessman, had started to decline from early dementia, and was getting depressed from his loss of function. Cheryl took him to the doctor who diagnosed his problem. When she returned home and shared the information with her mother, she became angry and told her husband he was no good to her for anything any longer. Cheryl herself was shocked and angry, but before she could comfort her father, he went to the bedroom. She heard the door lock and immediately thought her father might try to kill himself. In the next instant, she heard a loud noise. She rammed down the door and found him shot in the face. She called the paramedics and then tried to stop the bleeding. He lived until he got to the emergency room where he died of cardiac arrest. She witnessed horrors that are usually reserved for a battle scene. She had all of the classic symptoms of PTSD; hyper arousal, sleep disorder, flashbacks—all complicated by acute bereavement. I instituted immediate therapeutic intervention, and after acknowledging her loss, focused on her anger. The deep anger, which was addressed in our earlier work, had returned in spades. It now was further complicated by actual guilt and self-blame for not protecting her father from her mother's rage, and actual guilt for not anticipating her father's lethal action. She was furious with her mother, and that anger experience became the immediate focus. I was able to cleave the anxiety from the anger and her hyper arousal diminished. The next intervention dealt with her anger at her father for his subservience to her mother and, in fact, the proximate event prior to his suicide was her attack on his lack of value to her. Eventually she was able to forgive her father for his character flaw and, in so doing, freed herself from her dependency on cold and distant men. With resolution of her anger at her father, she herself dealt more effectively with her mother and told her mother about her anger for her mother's actions both immediate and long-term. The mother herself decided to enter psychotherapy, and their relationship survived and even improved. Six months after termination, Cheryl sent me a wedding announcement with a note that she was ready to accept real love from a man whom she described as warm, caring, supportive, and compassionate.

3. The Way Faulty Attachment is Transmitted from Generation to Generation

Modern attachment theory focuses on the process of attunement, which is largely a nonverbal, right hemispheric mode of communication between caregiver and child (Schore, 1997). Affect regulation through psychic and somatic mechanisms is of critical importance in healthy development. When the child and his environment are out of balance, and *no repair takes place,* small t trauma occurs, resulting in anger and eventually, defenses. What leads to a traumatized state of mind? The key ingredient seems to be a state of helplessness in the face of actual (or perceived) danger (Freud, 1926). Attunement failures between parent and child always are, by definition, small t traumas. If they are repetitive, fixed and rigid, there is no way to process the negative emotion that the trauma creates, and the effects become cumulative (Kahn, 1963). Ideally, small and even Big T traumatizing experiences are processed in the parent child dyad. However, when there is *impairment of parental empathy,* these affects are not processed interpersonally, they are stored. In an attempt to define trauma in a non-trivial way, Joseph Jones (1995, p. 116) explains, "a traumatized state occurs when a person is unable to respond appropriately to a situation; in turn, this inability to respond is signaled by anxiety-panic." Depending upon 1) the child's temperament, 2) the degree of the trauma, and 3) the capacity of the caregivers to respond, an insecure attachment may form. I have coined the term "primitive aggressive self-organization (PASO)" to describe this acquired form of insecure attachment. I will have more to say about this term later in the chapter. In the optimal parent child dyad, in Francine Shapiro's metaphor, the negative affects may be "digested" and no pathology results. Table 1 categorizes the types of traumas that patients bring with them to therapists in clinical practices.

Table 3. The Spectrum of Trauma: Conceptualization of Trauma: Small "t" as well as Big "T"

Parenting
Faulty attunement by either or both caregivers
Faulty empathy by either or both caregivers
Role Reversal by either or both caregivers
Faulty application of boundaries from caregivers
Favoritism; sibling rivalry
Neglect
Exploitative
Sexual abuse
Physical abuse
Power abuse: children as pawns (triangulation)
Environmental
Death of parent or sibling
Injury of person or body part
Divorce
Poverty
Natural disasters
Social discrimination: sex, race, cultural

I have chosen to present a patient whose core areas of conflict demonstrate how small t trauma can have major pathogenic effects on the development of mood and behavioral disorders. When preparing for this chapter, I considered presenting a patient with Big T trauma—one whose mother was psychotic and brutally beat both her and her sibling. This patient subsequently developed a life-threatening eating disorder. Ironically this less traumatic case that I will present below also resulted in a severe eating disorder. Again, Francine Shapiro's terminology, "Big T trauma," refers to the kind of experiences in DSM IV that cause posttraumatic stress disorder: catastrophic experiences outside the realm of ordinary experience. Small t trauma are those events in childhood that produce a sense of helpless, anxiety, shame, humiliation, and/or abandonment for which there has been no satisfactory repair from any caregiver. Much of this small t trauma is split off from consciousness and stored in largely inaccessible (nonlinguistic) form in the right hemisphere (Seigel, 1995, 1999). As I stressed earlier, Big T trauma inevitably activates dormant small t trauma.

It is my proposition that patients who are exposed to small t trauma (cumulative trauma, Kahn, 1963; Main, Main and Hesse, 1991, 1993, in press) develop an insecure attachment underling their mood and behavioral disorders. I believe that effective psychotherapeutic treatment can only occur when the patient faces the complex feelings that are "inside the insecure attachment." The resolution of successful psychotherapy means that the patient and therapist have created an "earned secure attachment." The secure attachment phenomenon is undoubtedly mediated by the neurotransmitters in the limbic system, and primarily serotonin, norepinephrine, and dopamine.[6] It is my opinion that much of psychopharmacology actually manipulates this system. Serotonin reuptake inhibitors ameliorate anxiety, decrease aggression and induce secure attachment phenomenon. In theory this is a wonderful thing, however, the effect may be largely "state dependent" and new learning often doesn't take place and unfortunately the patient remains dependent on the drug for freedom from depression and anxiety. On the other hand, many psychotherapies with

6. Acetylcholine is an important cortical neurotransmitter involved with affect regulation as well. It may mediate major defensive operation as well as shame, guilt and despair. (Neborsky and Janowsky, 1980)

these patients fail as well because the therapists lack either the technical or theoretical skill to overcome the patient's resistance to experiencing the feelings that exist inside the unconscious insecure attachment. Many therapies either do not address resistance or purport to address resistance but in fact do not overcome the barrier to genuine feeling. I frequently see patients who have had years of psychoanalysis and the core attachment pathology has not yielded even to this prolonged technique.

In *Short-Term Therapy for Long-Term Change,* I introduced the term "PASO" as a short-hand for the complex mixture of feelings and defenses that exist inside the insecure attachment. It is important to emphasize that these feelings are not conscious. They are highly conflicted and are either repressed or dissociated. It is my belief that all successful therapies restore the patient to a state of secure attachment, and their ability to experience contentment, to have joyful intimate relationships, to exert healthy self-assertion increases and they become resilient to stress-laden situations. Habib Davanloo (1995c) first described the "PASO"—without using the term—in his pioneering efforts to develop a short-term psychotherapy. Clinicians like myself who trained with Davanloo have developed our own spin-off therapies that rely on his original discoveries. The foundation of the short-term dynamic psychotherapies therapy lies in the belief that the patient must experience their *genuine feelings from the past in the present.* The transcript of a consultative interview with a patient with long-standing anxiety, depression and compulsive overeating will show how this is accomplished. In my work, I have added an important component to the goal of *genuine feelings from the past in the present*: I want the patient to leave their initial interview with a coherent narrative of the origin of their psychopathology. By a coherent narrative, I mean an understanding of the origins of their difficulties that includes the unconscious perspective. They will understand the dynamic origin of their anxiety, they will understand the role of anger, guilt and/or shame in their depression or self abuse.

They also will understand unconscious anger and its relationship to their other affects. These insights and understandings will be experiential as opposed to intellectual. In some cases, but not all, the inter-generational transmission of the trauma will become clear; however, all comprehensive treatments will trace the origin of their difficulties back to the grandparents.

In fact, patients receiving this treatment are freed from the unconscious transmission of the trauma to their children. Currently I am working on a series of cases where I have video-recorded "unlockings of the unconscious[7]" of parents and their adult neurotic children (Lifespan Learning Institute: Hysteria Conference, Los Angeles October 2000). The inter-generational transmission of unconscious trauma is startlingly apparent.

Now let's take a closer look at the PASO and see how it operates and then how I believe small t trauma is transferred from one generation to the next.

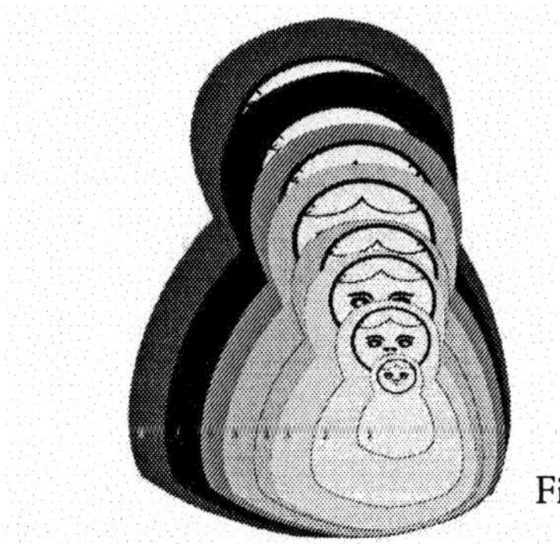

Figure 1. The "PASO"

I want to thank Marion Solomon (Co-author of *Short-Term Therapy for Long-Term Change*) for her illustration of the PASO and the idea of using Russian dolls. Let's examine the PASO in more detail.

9. At the center of the PASO (insecure attachment) lies *the capacity for secure attachment.* When this is present the individual has the capacity for contentment. Relationships are intimate and empathy for the feeling processes of others is intact.
10. Next, lies the emotion of *pain.* Classically, pain is not considered an emotion against which people defend. In our system it is. Herein we record the emotion of pain, and call it "pain of trauma."
11. Closely allied to pain is *sadness.* This is the sadness of loss of the closeness with the attachment figure.

---

7. A term invented by Davanloo (1995) to describe the process that I will present in the video.

12. In this level the *retaliatory rage* that is repressed in the unconscious can be found. This rage is frequently left unnoticed in traditional therapy. In Bowlby's (1973) model the existence of this rage for an extended period of time leads to despair.
13. *Anxiety* is found at this ring of the PASO that surrounds the sadness and/or the rage.
14. This level contains the *"crippling inhibitory affects"* of shame or guilt.
15. Overlaying the aforementioned affects are the defenses. There are several layers of *defenses: the tactical, the dynamic and the characterologic.*
16. Layer eight is seen only in more highly resistant cases: we call this the *defense against emotional closeness.* This is a defensive position in which detachment from all relatedness pervades the person's psyche.

Although I haven't schematized it, grief is also frequently encountered between the defenses and the guilt-shame layer. This sadness is a function of the lost time and opportunities the patient has suffered from the existence of their defenses. Sexual feeling is located between layers four and five. Sexuality and aggressive feeling can be commingled when certain types of abuse and empathic failures occur.

Short-term dynamic psychotherapy explores this structure in each and every psychotherapy session. The way this is done varies with different styles of short-term therapy. But all short-term therapies focus on the patient's resistance (defenses) and techniques are used to overcome those defenses. It is the defenses that interfere with the patient's ability to process painful affects and restore a healthy operative self. Francine Shapiro has demonstrated beyond any doubt that experience of affect is more essential to cure than is interpretation. In Dr. Shapiro's (1995, 2001) model of therapy, the therapist's job is to give the brain the opportunity to process affective-laden information in a safe atmosphere. She emphasizes the neutrality of the therapist and stresses the brain's inherent ability to process traumatic information and to develop a positive solution. EMDR allows dissociated and repressed affects to become conscious and to be "re-processed." Short-term dynamic psychotherapy operates in much the same way. The cure is promoted by the patient's ability to access the emotions described in the PASO—layers 1 through 6.

I want to focus on two particular aspects of the unconscious for the purposes of this volume. One is the intergenerational transmission of trauma (Ainsworth, 1991), and the other is compulsive behavior. Mary Main (1991, 1993, in press) has discussed data that shows that psychopathology can be predicted in children of mothers with an incoherent narrative. The incoherent narrative is thought to reflect unresolved trauma in the mother. Mothers with unresolved trauma defend against the affects that are mobilized in that area of trauma. However, that trauma which is not processed is repeated in behavior. The mothers in effect treat their children the same way they themselves were treated.

The patient in this presentation was overly controlled by her mother, as was her mother by her grandmother. The sad loss was the loss of mutuality of joyful interchange between mother and child. Further compounding the problem in this particular case, the patient was made to feel responsible (reinforcement of unconscious omnipotence) for the mother's illness and heart condition. The child began to feel angry with the mother, and neither mother nor grandmother could tolerate the child's anger. The child's anger developed in intensity and power. The intensity of the anger became associated with death wishes toward the mother. The mother's real illness compounded the fear (anxiety) over the death wishes. The patient loved her mother and began to feel guilty not only over her angry feelings toward mother but also the "real" damage her existence caused her mother (high blood pressure, heart attack, stress). Next, the mother, who in some way found her child to be a burden, became embroiled in a power struggle with the daughter over food intake. (This most likely represents a re-enactment of a power struggle with mother's mother). Food soon became a weapon with which the patient could express negative autonomy, and a way in which the child could passive-aggressively express anger against mother and also relieve guilt through punishment of self.

Over time, the patient naturally begins to grow, develop and separate and individuate. However, the damage was already done (Stroufe, 1990). Her self-regulatory processes are disordered. Her attachment has turned from potentially secure to insecure avoidant with a fully developed

PASO. Another way of thinking about this issue is that she has failed to separate and individuate in a positive frame. Instead she is always with the mother who suppressed her joyful side and she is full of unconscious anger directed now not outwardly against mother, but against herself. The guilt over the rage against mother is continuously undone by self-abuse. The more she can destroy her health, the less guilty, and the less anxious she feels.

What, one might ask, drives this process over years and years, and why doesn't the patient just learn new behaviors? The answer is, she can't. First the information she needs to unlearn is split-off into non-verbal right hemisphere memory. The process is driven by the propensity for transference, projection and projective identification with authority figures in her life. It is eerie and hard to acknowledge but there is a powerful unconscious force in trauma patients called narrative re-enactment (Vander Kolk, 1989). Freud (1918) recognized it, as did Erik Erikson (1963) as did Davanloo (Oral communication). So the patient is driven to attach herself to figures that resemble her mother and grandmother so she can re-enact the original trauma. The reasons behind this are controversial. Davanloo believes that the compulsion to repeat is a superego phenomenon to punish the self over and over again for the unconscious anger at the offending relative. Earlier theorists like Freud (1911, 1926) and Erikson (1963) saw it as an attempt to master the trauma. It is probably a combination of both, particularly in patients who present for therapy.

In my opinion, the compulsive behavior serves another function as well. Since there is no internal, stable secure attachment the patient has to rely on external sources for stability. Her feelings themselves are not a secure place. Compulsion is predictable, stable and reliable—albeit rigid, and mal-adaptive. It is also self destructive in that overeating and bulimia can result in an actual death of the self. Therefore the compulsive behavior compensates for the missing capacity to support and soothe oneself in the face of adversity.

4. The Technique of Treating Attachment Trauma

The therapeutic approach that I have adopted is modeled after the use of the Central Dynamic Sequence.

Table 4. The Central Dynamic Sequence

	Phase	*Task*
1	Inquiry	Gathering areas of disturbance; exploring the difficulties; initial ability to respond
2	Pressuring toward feeling	Leads to resistance in the form of defenses; rapid identification of the character defenses; clarification and challenge to the defenses; psychodiagnosis
3	Challenging resistances	Challenge combined with a lack of respect for resistances; crystallization of the character resistances; application of partial head–on collision to show resistance has paralyzed his functioning and turn patient against his resistance
4	Transference resistances	Mounting challenge to transference resistance; intensify rise in transference feelings; mobilize the therapeutic alliance against the resistance; loosen the psychic system
5	Direct access to the unconscious	Intrapsychic crisis; breakthrough of complex transference feelings; direct view of the psychopathologic forces responsible for the patient's symptom and character disturbance
6	Analysis of the transference	Summarize the I/F-A-D-character system just experienced in the transference in order to resole residual resistance
7	Dynamic exploration into the unconscious	Now the unconscious therapeutic alliance is in control of the process; patient spontaneously introduces traumatic events; repeated breakthroughs of guilt and grief laden feelings; consolidation recapitulation and psychotherapeutic plan

The term "Central Dynamic Sequence" was coined by collaboration between David Malan and Davanloo in the 1960s and 70s. They studied a large population of six hundred patients with a broad spectrum of psychoneurotic and characterologic difficulties. The techniques within this system were developed from a combination of creative inspiration and simple trial and error—evaluated with videotape for effectiveness. The results of that impressive research effort were never formally published, but anecdotally 80% of the patients showed dramatic improvement.)

Table 5.

Techniques used in Short-term Dynamic Psychotherapy
1. Maintaining a focus
2. Pressure toward feeling
3. Clarifying the experience of feeling, defense, and anxiety
4. Challenging the use of defenses as self harming
5. Confrontation with the consequences of maintaining defense or characterologic habits to avoid feeling
6. Body experiencing of the core emotions
7. Visualization of the action tendency of each felt emotion in the now
8. Linking of the emotions with events or important figures from the past
9. Affective repair through closeness with the emotions of the therapist

Davanloo's research suggests that the healing process is facilitated if the patient can experience the feelings "underneath" the anxiety or depression with which the patient presents. The therapeutic process starts with a survey of the patient's areas of disturbance: symptoms and relational problems. After this information is gathered, the patient and the therapist begin to explore a single incident wherein the patient experienced anxiety: this can be in their current life or in the transference in the here and now. I then proceed with psycho-education about what Malan and Davanloo called the "Triangle of Conflict" (1990). The goal is to get the patient to recognize the presence of unconscious affect present in the room, and how that affect is creating problems. Furthermore the patient is educated about the defense mechanisms, which he or she is using to contain these affects. Next, the patient is shown how these defenses, albeit useful at one time, are now harmful, and must be relinquished in order for the treatment to work. The goal then becomes the experience of unconscious emotion, free of anxiety and free of defense. In order to accomplish this, the patient must ally with the therapist and create what Davanloo has called an unconscious therapeutic alliance.

Usually there is an encounter with raw, un-neutralized aggression, deep grief, guilt, and/or shame. The process then opens the unhealed wounds of past trauma for direct inspection by the patient, and the therapist. The underlying feelings of the original trauma are made conscious, and through the therapist's attunement and empathy, the therapeutic repair occurs. The emotions are worked through with the utilization of visualization and trance, which offers possibilities for repair. Self-destructive behavior patterns dissipate, and the patient develops self directed compassion, and empathy for others, including the offending parental figure. The patient and therapist terminate the relationship when the working through is complete, and presenting symptoms and/or character disturbances are gone.

5. Edited Transcript of Six Hours of Attachment-Based Psychotherapy

Clinical Case 3: Insecure Attachment: No Big T Trauma, Complete Resolution of Small t Trauma.

The Woman Who Pleased Too Much

The patient is a forty-five-year old married woman who works as an assistant for a insurance executive. She has a long history of eating disorders, including bulimia. Her therapist, Sharon, referred her to Dr. Neborsky for a consultation to assist with her ongoing therapy. Dr. Neborsky begins this first session by asking the patient to define her areas of disturbance.

P: I've battled weight most of my life. I have a history of bulimia. Um, I haven't purged in years now . . . and I seem to be stuck with getting to whatever it is that is having me hold on to the weight.

T: Uh-huh.

P: You know, whatever it is that I'm using that for, um, I've had some definite positive shifts with Sharon. I'm a lot less unwilling to make myself uncomfortable with food in the time I'm eating. But the thing that I'm really aware of is that I'm uncomfortable on a daily basis. You know, sitting in this chair right now, I'm really . . . everything feels in the way.

It's hard to sit in a way that my back doesn't hurt. So I can't pretend that I'm not bothered by my weight . . .

T: Uh-huh.

P: And yet, I seem to keep eating in a way that is keeping me fat.

T: What do you do?

P: I don't diet. Um, I kind of struggle . . . with, um, I'm about to cry . . . I think I've struggled with the fear that to start dieting again will lead to bulimia again.

T: Hum, so there's a painful memory of the days when you had bulimia?

P: Yeah, and I think that I'm afraid that if I can't use the discipline that it sometimes takes to lose the weight that I will start caring too much again . . . (cries)

T: Umm.

P: And that, uh . . .

T: So you're actually keeping yourself detached from part of your feelings . . . in order to not care.

P: Yeah, yeah, you're right.

T: Now, let's get off the weight topic for just a moment—are there any other areas that you're aware of where there are problems, uh, that we should focus our attention on while we're together here?

P: Um, I have a feeling that if I'm not perfect, I won't be loved.

T: Hum.

P: And I've become aware of that, and can kind of talk myself through that a lot, but, um, it's still kind of in that phase of I'm aware of it as its happening and I'm able to say, "No, this is your old stuff." You know, this is not real . . . this is your projection, but, uh . . .

T: Wait. You're describing fear, aren't you? . . . there's a considerable amount of fear . . . there's two sides of it.

P: (Crying) Yeah . . . yeah, I never thought of it as fear, but that's exactly what it feels like.

T: Now, any other areas? Let's keep on going down the inventory of things, you know, that you're concerned about, or anything you'd like.

P: Um . . . (long pause) Hm . . . I don't know where . . . what I'm supposed to . . .

T: Well, we've talked about, you know, not modifying or modulating your diet because of fear.

P: Uh-huh.

T: We talked about this way you have of trying to stay out of fear by trying to be perfect in order to ensure love . . . anything else? Any depression? Any . . .

P: Um, yeah, depression.

T: Tell me about that, the history . . .

P: Um, I'm think when it started . . . I think I was depressed as a teenager and my mother had had a heart attack when I was in the 6th grade. And so I kind of grew up with the stress of, um, thinking that if I did something wrong that she'd die . . . because if she'd get upset, it would raise her blood pressure. This is a conversation my father had, that I shouldn't argue with my mother because if she got really upset and her blood pressure got high, she might have another heart attack and die. (Laughs.) After years of therapy, I can see the humor in that . . .

T: Uh-huh.

P: And how I couldn't make her die.

T: But that would put fear in you, wouldn't it?

P: Oh, definitely. (Cries.)

T: You know, every time I mention fear, you start to cry . . .

P: Yeah, I do!

T: What's that about? I mean, what do you experience?

P: I think it's the first time that I've ever thought of the word 'fear' . . .

T: In all the therapy?

P: Well, but it's the first time that I've ever thought about it as a big issue.

T: Uh-huh.

P: And I think I'm just getting that it really is a big issue. Just talking about it, I live a lot of my life afraid.

T: Uh-huh.

P: I'm just remembering what it was like to have a mother who's always sick . . . that I was always afraid was going to die . . . (cries).

T: Would you share that memory with me?

P: I can remember like coming home from school and feeling anxious about whether or not she was going to be OK when I walked in, you know, and had to be really careful when I had friends over . . . to make sure they're not going to tell her things that I thought might make her upset.

T: Uh-huh.

P: I'm thinking about a memory of being in the 4th grade and making a B+ in math. My parents both taught algebra.

T: Uh-huh.

P: And my mother yelled at me for 45 minutes, just raged about it. I felt really shamed and uncomfortable and abused. (Laughs.) And, uh, I don't know, I just associate that a lot to . . . it's not like I made a B+ in math on purpose, you know. I mean, I was supposed to make all A's . . .

T: I'm not sure what you're telling me here. It's important. You see, it's coming in a little bit of a jumble. Are you telling me a story about a way you were being abused? Is that the story?

P: I think that's the story, but also why it became so important to be perfect, and why I became so fearful . . . (cries) . . . of trying things . . . of failing . . .

T: Fear of failure—because you would be abused if you didn't meet perfection?

P: I think that love is more the word that . . .

T: Well, you were scolded, I mean, that's pretty severe . . . thirty minutes of rage.

P: Yeah, yeah.

T: Was this before or after your mother had the heart attack?

P: Before (cries).

T: You're crying . . . you're expressing something . . . what's going on?

P: Oh, sadness, I think.

T: I think so, too. Sadness related to what?

P: (Sighs.)

T: The relationship related to your mom?

P: Yeah . . . and being treated that way. You know . . .

T: What was your emotional reaction? You had mentioned shame.

P: Anger . . . I was really angry. I just remember going up to my room and crying on my bed for a few hours.

T: So you wept in the face of anger?

P: Yeah (sighs).

T: What was that sigh about?

P: (Laughs) It just felt good. It's like a deep breath . . .

T: Can you remember, as you sit here, your anger specifically? Do you have a specific memory of it? How it felt?

P: Yeah. I remember one incident . . . I mean . . . (punches arms in air) I feel it here; like shoulders (touches shoulders), and punching kinds of feelings . . .

T: Uh-huh. But you didn't do that?

P: No—no.

The patient describes how, in a session with her therapist, Sharon, she fantasized killing her mother by severing her head.

T: You wept instead.

P: Uh-huh.

T: So the weakness was in being abandoned on the one hand, but it was also a defense against the more angry part of the feeling.

T: A question comes to mind, of course, when you did that, what were your feelings? What was your reaction?

P: I felt really calm . . . it felt really good. It felt like a real release . . .

T: I'm confused about something—I don't understand why when you really did have the opportunity to kill your mother, you acted so fearful.

P: I don't understand—what do you mean?

T: Well, didn't you tell me after your mom had a heart attack . . .

P: Oh, right . . .

T: That your dad told you that if you did anything to upset her, she'd die?

P: Uh-huh.

T: What stopped you from . . .

P: I didn't want her to die.

T: Well, tell me about that. What's that all about?

P: Uh . . . (long pause).

T: See, in the murder fantasy, there was a part of you that wanted her to die . . .

P: Right, but that was like as an adult, like in the last year, that thing that I did with Sharon. I didn't do that as a child.

T: So you didn't have the same feelings when you were a child?

P: I probably did, but I . . . well, I don't know . . . I don't know if I just censored them. You know, I mean, you aren't supposed to kill people, you know? I was raised in a Presbyterian church and went to Sunday school every Sunday, and you weren't supposed to kill people and weren't supposed to wish people were dead.

T: What did that make you, if you did?

P: You'd go to hell . . . (laughs) . . . nothing to be afraid of with that one, just burn there for the rest of eternity . . . I mean, I don't believe in that stuff anymore, but . . . (laughs).

T: But, wouldn't there be a reason for going to hell?

P: Well, yeah, for the sin of wanting your mother to be dead. I don't know. I keep waiting for you to say something. I'm not sure . . . it seems so clear to me.

T: It seems clear to me, too, but it also doesn't seem to me that you're putting 2 + 2 together.

P: I don't know what you mean.

T: Well, the feelings of wanting your mother to be dead, according to you, is a sin and according to you, the way you're taught, you should go to hell and burn.

P: Uh-huh.

T: So you committed a sin, right?

P: Uh-huh.

T: So what's the punishment for the sin, for wanting her dead?

P: I don't know if I wanted her dead then. I think . . .

T: When did she yell at you?

P: When I was in the 4th grade. I'm not following you . . .

T: Didn't you just show me all the anger? You know, I'm putting this all together for you, what you've done with Sharon, right? In other words, you said you had all of these murder feelings with your mom and they came out in therapy with Sharon. You knocked your mom's block off and after you knocked her block off, you stomped on her head.

P: Uh-huh.

T: There's no doubt. She's dead.

P: Right.

T: The only question here is when those feelings began.

P: Oh, I see . . . (pause) . . . Well, they probably began before that, but that's the first, like memory, I'm attaching it to.

T: OK, so . . . what's the punishment?

P: The punishment? To me?

T: Yeah, to you. (Long pause.) It seems pretty clear and simple to me . . . its true and simple . . . to live in perpetual fear.

P: Oh, (laughs) it wasn't clear to me at all.

T: It's easy, (laughs). I'm sitting here in this chair, and you're sitting there . . .

P: Yeah . . . Wow . . . (cries). Yeah, that's interesting . . . because there's been so many things like that. I have this fear about me causing other people to suffer. And I have a fear when I'm driving, I mean not a paralyzing fear, but, you know (sighs), I've had the thought is the clearest way to put it, that how horrible it would be if you accidentally ran over somebody with an automobile. You know, how would you live with yourself if you knew you caused another person's death? Wow . . .

T: Like?

P: Like, if I had done that to my mother . . . (cries). Wow . . . even to the point of just hurting somebody's feelings inadvertently. Just saying something that you don't mean to hurt another person's feelings, and you realize that you have or, I mean, I'll worry about something I said to somebody, and think, gee, you know, I'll almost obsess over, oh, I hope they don't think I meant this . . .

T: Trying to undo the deed, spending you time undoing it, which you may or may not have done?

P: Yeah, yeah, exactly . . . and working with Sharon, I've come out of projecting a lot of that, but I'm now seeing that that's the same thing.

T: So what feelings are you now relating to? What emotions are you describing?

P: Well, I think fear . . .

T: Well, it's a combination . . . I think there' some guilt.

P: Oh, and guilt.

T: Yeah . . .

P: Yeah, guilt. (Laughs.) Oh, I finally get it, it's like, oh, duh, guilt!

T: Yeah, but it's important. Actually, you've been very quick. But I think, like you've been saying—organization—I don't think you're putting together all of the pieces of the psychological puzzle into a coherent whole . . . so that you can see that you've had all of these murderous feelings toward your mom as a child, and you lived in a tremendous amount of fear that those murderous feelings would come true, and you feel guilty about having those murderous feelings . . . right?

P: (Cries.) Yeah!

T: And the punishment is to, you know, live in one of the outer rings of hell, which is perpetual fear.

P: (Cries.) Wow.

T: You know, fear, paralysis . . . and really in the sense, almost paralyzed to take positive action on your own behalf.

P: Yeah, absolutely . . . fear about my parents who had me when they were forty-five, and they had not planned to have a third child. And so, um, I knew that, oh boy (laughs), I knew that they had not planned to have a third child and that's when my mother's health problems started, with her pregnancy, and that's when she started having high blood pressure, and they actually wanted to give her an abortion . . . and that was forty-five years ago when they just didn't do that . . . it would have been a medical abortion because of the blood pressure and her kidneys and things like that . . .

T: What did you say . . . 'wow'?

P: Because I got this . . . went even back that far . . . the guilt about causing . . . the fear . . . causing her to die . . . that was already out there before I was even born. The whole thought of . . . of, it's like before I was even born, I was causing her to die. Wow, that's pretty big! (Sniffs.) I'm surprised . . . (pause) I'm surprised I'm not seven hundred pounds! (Laughs.)

T: That was an amazing connection, wasn't it?

P: Yeah. (Laughs.)

T: What was the connection?

P: Just the whole thing that I've grown up with all the pressure and guilt and self-punishment. It's amazing that, you know, that I haven't created an even more uncomfortable body . . .

T: . . . in which to torture yourself, make yourself uncomfortable . . .

P: Yeah . . . the outer ring of hell.

T: Uh-huh, and guilt over your, um, destroying your mother just based on your own life, your own creation. Nothing that you did or didn't do . . . just your own struggle to survive.

P: Yeah (nods).

T: See, so you use food as a weapon, really, to destroy yourself.

P: Yep. Wow. I know that intellectually, and then get it, and it's . . .

T: Get it *emotionally.* Tell me, what's that like? What happens if you let that sink in?

P: (Long pause.) It's to make the conscious choice of . . . it feels like . . . it feels like there's the option of a conscious choice not to do that. To make, to realize that you don't really need to do this to yourself (long pause). I'm feeling like I could do it, like I could quit doing this . . . and that feels good.

T: Uh-huh, see can you understand now in a deeper fashion the relationship between dieting and bulimia. See, it seems to me that if you're not using one weapon—food—to kill yourself, then you have to substitute and use the bulimia as your secret weapon to hurt yourself.

P: Yeah, because I've never really believed that I deserved to be on the planet. It's like I know it in my mind, but not on a gut level. (Cries.) Because it was like I grew up believing that I was this big, horrible inconvenience to my parents, and that my mother almost died because of me.

T: Do you have any memory at all of any time blaming yourself for your mother's heart attack?

P: (Cries, nods yes.) The night she had the heart attack was the night of our band banquet and she wasn't feeling well. I was in the band and I had been nominated as the most outstanding band student that year. And we were having a banquet that night and awards were going to be given out, and she didn't feel well and didn't want to go and I kind of pushed and pushed, until she went. And she actually had her heart attack at the band banquet. (Cries.) And we went straight to our family doctor's house from the banquet and he called an ambulance and took her to the hospital. She'd had a very serious heart attack.

T: OK, talk, talk the emotions. What you're feeling, tell me about that . . .

P: Guilty! (Cries.) Wow! And at some point later, she told me I had caused her heart attack.

T: So she confirmed it!

P: Yeah.

T: It really seems to me that in part you've taken on this struggle, and you truthfully are trying to induce an illness in yourself. In other words, If you get a heart attack, then it seems to me the debt is, in part, repaid.

P: Wow! (Cries.) Yeah. I have a good life . . . after ruining hers.

T: So it seems to me that if we really get down to the bottom of the issue, guilt is the major engine of your difficulties, creating this kind of like dilemma you're in where you have to sabotage your efforts to stay healthy. I mean, you see that you're between a rock and a hard place?

P: Yes, I really do, and that's the perfect way to describe how it's felt for a while. It's like on this one hand, wanting to do it but on this other hand, not being able to do it. You know, I've been conscious about resistance about doing that. It's not even like . . . I can't pretend even to myself. It's like, oh, I really want to do it and I'm really trying my best . . . I know

I'm not. You know, I know, I've been conscious that I've actually resisted doing . . .

T: So its sabotage . . .

P: Yeah.

T: You see what I mean?

P: Yeah, I totally do.

T: With your help.

P: Uh-huh. And, in fact, when people would notice that I'm losing weight, and I always thought this was because I got so tired of being noticed for losing weight.

T: Well, the mind can work in tricky ways . . . I mean, you may be right, who knows, I wasn't there. But I can give you another spin on it . . . that life was going too good, and you were getting too much glory, and too much recognition, and too much admiration, and then the forces of self-sabotage began to undermine your own thinking, right? And made that the problem! Rather than the unconscious guilt of having a good life after all this stuff with your mom, both the guilt of your very birth, your very creation, you know, causing her harm, and then secondarily, this controlling part of your mom that would suppress your natural instincts. She would just sort of push down the joyous part of you, right? And that makes you very shameful and very angry.

P: (Nods, cries.)

T: And then you would wish harm to her, and then harm happens to her, and then you're dead in the water. And then you have this guilt that you carry with you for the rest of your life. It's huge. Much bigger than your weight problem.

The patient recalls an incident in which she was angry at her boss, Roger. She admits to having "pushed down" her anger and asks the therapist if there is a "right way" of expressing it. Dr. Neborsky answers that it's necessary, first, to experience the anger and asks, "How did your anger feel?"

P: My ears were ringing and, um, I felt nauseous . . . my heart was racing.

T: I'm just pointing out to you again . . . you know . . . I'm not blaming you for this, I'm just describing so that you can learn. You're turning your anger against your own body, aren't you?

P: Yeah.

T: Ringing ears, nausea, you're turning the anger against you.

P: Wow, so that's not how most people feel? I mean . . . I just thought that that was . . . wow!

T: That's how people feel anger that's turned inward. Ringing ears and nausea . . .

P: So you can have anger and not those feelings? I don't think I've ever had it (cries). It never even occurred to me that you could have anger and not have those feelings.

T: That's anger turned inward, right?

P: I get it.

T: Do you remember the muscular-skeletal part of the anger?

P: Yeah, I was very tense. I was gripping and all that stuff . . .

T: Uh-huh, so you were having an impulse.

P: Uh, oh, I get it, yeah. I was holding back an impulse to go punch his brains out.

T: That was it?

P: Yeah, that's it, I wasn't having an impulse, I was holding it back.

T: I know.

P: Wow.

T: Can you capture the impulse you were holding back? (Pause.) When you think it through carefully, what's the impulse?

P: Just scream at him . . .

T: Lash out verbally. OK.

P: Uh-huh.

T: OK, but remember, see that's to leave the stressful situation. The impulse is in your arms. That simple. Impulse isn't so much verbal as it is physical. Physical rises when the heart is beating, blood is rushing through your body, right? Because of the rapid heartbeat, that's the anger response. You cut that anger off by turning it out against Mary (pause) with the nausea and ringing in the ears. So keep your mind's eye focused on the body, on your body.

P: Uh-huh.

T: Expressing the impulse . . . what would it look like? If you lost control, and you know that I know you never will, but if you did lose control in that room . . .

P: Oh, I would then jump up to my feet and run toward him, and put my hands around his neck and start shaking him. I would have slapped his face. I would have pulled out his hair implants, and I would have picked him up and swung him around by his hair, and just slammed him against the mirrors, and slammed him against the stereo, and slammed him against the floor . . . in front of everybody. And just slammed him around the room and then, just, just, um . . . (pause) thrown him on the floor and jumped on him . . . just jumped up and down with both feet (pause).

T: Would he survive . . . that kind of assault? (Long silence.) If you looked at his eyes, what would you see in his eyes?

P: Fear . . . shock . . . um . . .

T: Pain?

P: Yeah (nods).

T: And what would you like him to be thinking?

P: I better stop this behavior (pause). I was wrong (pause) . . .

T: To use force and coercion and shame . . . against you . . .

P: Uh-huh, uh-huh.

T: Would he survive? That was my question.

P: Yeah, he would survive. I would want him to survive. I don't know if he'd survive if I was jumping up and down on him, I mean, its indescribable what I'd do to him.

T: See the conflict? The anger is so strong that he wouldn't survive, but the heart—the love wants him to survive.

P: Wow (nods).

T: So tell me, in the scenario where he doesn't survive, with the anger so big that he doesn't survive the assault?

P: Where in the scenario?

T: If you were jumping on his chest, causing him to die . . .

P: Oh, I get it, it would be breaking limbs and puncturing lungs . . .

T: OK, we know that stuff, but what would your reaction be, how would you respond when you came to your senses?

P: (Pause.) I would be really sad.

T: What would you do?

P: Try to save him.

T: How?

P: I'd call 911. I'd start CPR. I'd try to stop . . . try to control the bleeding . . .

T: And when you realized it was to no avail? . . .

P: Well, I'd probably kill myself! (Long pause.) (Nods.) Wow. (Long pause.) Yeah (shakes head), I'd feel so guilty, I wouldn't be able to live with that.

T: So killing yourself would be your way of undoing the crime of killing Roger?

P: Uh-huh. (Long pause.) Hum.

T: Hum, what?

P: Its just amazing to see all this—just amazing—so clearly right now and just see this thing that just goes throughout . . . the anger, that leads to the guilt, that leads to the fear, that leads to the self-destruction, that leads to . . . the self-destruction! (Laughs.) That's pretty much where it stops.

The patient returns the next day and says she has never considered her emotions to be genuine experiences. Dr. Neborsky asks the patient to make it a priority not to shut down her emotions, no matter how intense they may become.

P: I don't know if I know how.

T: I think you're aware that this is called the helpless position. You're taking helpless positions, and don't know how not to shut down . . . where will that get us?

P: Nowhere.

T: That's the self-sabotage. The first time in the session that self-sabotage is starting to show its head, so to speak, you nod "uh-huh." See the compliance? See, you're showing compliance, aren't you, but it's really pseudo-compliance because nothing's really happening. Why are you smiling?

P: I'm trying so hard to understand (touches head), but I know that's not what we're trying to do . . .

T: But I think you do understand . . . you see, it's not about understanding, Mary, it's about action. You shut down in the face of anxiety. Anxiety rises inside your whole being . . .

P: Uh-huh.

T: Your mouth gets dry . . .

P: Uh-huh . . . it feels like I've got butterflies in my stomach.

T: That's pure anxiety, isn't it?

P: Uh-huh . . .

T: No question about it, and your habit has been that when you get anxious, to shut down feelings and to go to intellect. And you understand that doing the same thing with me, you know, is silly because it's going to give you the same result. When you leave, see, that's what I mean by self-sabotage. If you go to your habits when you're here in the therapy session with me, all you do is reinforce the habits. So that sabotages new learning, doesn't it?

P: Yeah, it does (nods).

T: I mean when you leave here, it doesn't feel like you've gotten anything out of this session. You won't feel. You won't feel as though you've gotten as much out of the session, perhaps, as you felt you did yesterday.

P: Uh-huh.

T: And I don't want that to happen.

P: Right (nods).

T: But I've got to get you to recognize what your habits are. Instead of nodding like the compliant child, to take some action against the habit, to get in new habits. Because you just nod and go through these motions of pleasing me and you get nowhere.

P: (Nods, pause)

T: So what are you going to do about that wall that shuts down against those feelings that scare you? Because that's what anxiety is, a form of internalized fear. So your feelings are scaring you. They're creating anxiety. Mary is shutting down and you're going into your people-pleasing mode . . . with me. But that doesn't work. You see that?

P: Uh-huh.

T: So what are you going to do? (Silence) . . . about the shutting down, about the helplessness, about the people-pleasing façade?

P: (Nods)

T: Now, you're doing it again!

P: (Smiles, nods.) Right.

T: You smiled though and that indicates that you're covering the feeling or something. You're having a reaction, or you wouldn't be smiling if you weren't.

P: It's because I keep switching to here (touches head). I'm nodding at, OK, I'm in touch with what you're saying, you know.

T: But you see, that gets you nowhere . . .

P: I know . . .

T: And that's not going to cut the mustard, is it?

P: But I don't know what to do . . .

T: You see, see how its entrenched? You see, now you're becoming helpless . . .

P: (Laughs.)

T: Look at you. You're nodding when I tell you you're helpless. You see there's no action against these defenses, which are the source of your difficulties, which are what's keeping you stuck . . . obviously, which are three defenses . . .

P: The defenses being?

T: Helplessness, shutting down, right? And being a people-pleaser. We've got like these three core defenses.

P: (Softly) Being a people-pleaser . . . shutting down . . . and helplessness . . .

T: In the face of this anxiety, right?

P: Uh-huh.

T: Those are defenses against anxiety.

P: (Nods.) Uh-huh.

T: You're doing it again . . . you're nodding at me, but nothing's happening. You're not taking action against your defenses. So what are you going to do?

P: (Sighs deeply.)

T: You're shutting down . . . did you see the rise of anxiety in your body? (Imitates sigh.) You start getting anxious and that's the shutting down response, isn't it?

P: I think of that as a getting in touch thing . . .

T: I don't understand, what do you mean?

P: Its just like, OK, clear your mind and be quiet a second and feel . . .

T: OK, well that could be really positive . . .

P: Uh-huh.

T: But what I was also seeing is ignoring a rise in your anxiety. You're nodding . . . because I would hope that you would recognize that you're becoming more anxious. Did you recognize it?

P: Uh-uh (shakes head no).

T: Yes, see, I have the sense that what you're doing is self-hypnosis or self-relaxation . . . in the face of anxiety.

P: I've never thought of that.

T: It's a bona fide technique, OK?

P: Uh-huh.

T: OK, but I think I can perhaps offer you a better way . . .

P: OK, good.

T: But you'll have to endure the anxiety.

P: (Nods)

T: Do you follow me? You'd have to identify it for what it is.

P: You mean the physical feelings that I'm feeling?

T: Absolutely.

P: Well, I feel like I can't breathe as well . . . My palms are feeling real sweaty and my throat feels tight (touches throat). I have feelings in here (rubs stomach), lots of little butterfly feelings in here . . . a little nauseous. Shoulders feel tight (touches shoulders). My neck feels tight (touches neck).

T: That's an exquisite description of anxiety. Now, just stay in touch with that experience without defending against it. (Pause.)

P: What if I throw up? (Cries.) I think I'm crying because of the fear.

T: I'm not sure; I wouldn't jump to any conclusions about that. It can be very confusing, I mean you could be having a tremendous breakthrough of sadness.

P: (Cries.) This whole feeling of throwing up is about bulimia, you know, it's like . . .

T: I hear what you're saying, but be careful, OK, let's not make more into sadness than what it is. Nausea can be a symptom of anxiety. It can just be a symptom. I'm sure you have a memory bank about associations of throwing up.

P: Oh, no, I'm just saying that this sadness makes me think about the bulimia.

T: OK, good, but I think that that's a deflection that the sadness is the issue—that is the feeling that wants to come up . . . if you look at it like I do.

P: Yeah, right . . . (Sobs long time.)

T: And truly, feeling this sadness is the cure for the anxiety.

P: (Nods, sobs.)

T: There's waves of it, isn't there? It's like a wave.

P: (Nods, sobs.)

T: Another wave coming?

P: (Nods, sobs.)

T: Is there any thought with this sad feeling . . . just anything that comes into your thoughts?

P: My mother did . . . why couldn't I have had parents who were healthy . . . and loving . . . and that stuff, you know?

T: How, I mean, does that come into your thoughts?

P: It just flashed, it just flashed.
T: Uh-huh, so these are longings . . . for a very close relationship . . .
P: (Nods, cries.)
T: Its really painful . . . the longing for the closeness . . .
P: (Nods, cries.)
T: Let it come into . . . come into your mind as to what it was that you would have liked.
P: For her to like me . . .
T: And what would that entail in your imagination? Can you remember?
P: Um, she would not have squelched the things I loved to do . . . she would have encouraged me to do the things that I was good at and loved to do . . . she wouldn't have done the raging that she did . . . she wouldn't have blamed me for her health problems . . . (long pause) that's the only stuff that's coming out . . .
T: Uh-huh.
P: She would have wanted me to be born.

The patient recalls her maternal grandmother, a strict, critical woman. The patient felt that in her relationship with her grandmother she was "always walking on eggshells." Dr. Neborsky asks if there was ever any tenderness between the two of them.

P: (Shakes head.) I don't remember love and affection (long pause) . . . (shakes head).
T: What?
P: My eyes just felt dry. It was like all of a sudden, I was just going to fall asleep. (Laughs.)
T: Why?
P: I don't know.
T: Wouldn't that be cutting off feelings?
P: Probably. (Nods, cries.) (Long pause.) Oh, I hated going there . . . I was always afraid of her . . . (deep breaths). But I feel sad because a grandmother is supposed to love you . . . and bake you cookies . . . and give you milk, and . . . instead of . . .
T: Instead of what?
P: Instead of being mean to you and not wanting you around or making you feel that way . . . like a burden.
T: Hum, and your grandmother?

P: . . . it's so sad . . . (cries).

T: It's terribly sad, of course it is . . . your grandmother was dismissive as well as controlling towards your mother . . .

P: (Nods.) Yeah. (Cries.) I was sad for my mother, too, growing up with her . . . (Cries.) (Pause.)

T: Could you just elaborate on that some?

P: Well, she was the victim (?), too. And it makes me angry that she grew up with her, so how could she do that to me?

T: That's the way I see it (pause). In other words, if we could just summarize what you just said, your grandmother made your mother feel as though she was a burden, and your mother had some similar issues inside of her that she then transferred those issues to you.

P: Un-huh. (Nods.)

T: Making you feel as though your birth was a burden . . .

P: (Nods.)

T: And that raising you was a burden . . . just like her mom made her feel.

P: Yeah. (Nods.)

T: So it's kind of a three-generational disturbance . . .

P: Yeah, and I think that's one of the reasons I decided not to have children myself (cries).

T: Go on, tell me about that.

P: I was just afraid that I'd be like them . . .

T: Even in spite of all your fear therapy?

P: (Cries, nods.)

T: Tell me about that, I would like to understand . . .

P: Well, I'm not sure that's the only reason I decided not to have kids, but I just . . . because of the anxiety that I feel . . . and all the people-pleasing, and the anxiety . . . like when I have a warped-out (?) mind or something like that. I just have a feeling that I would be short and not give my children what they needed.

T: Well, I can understand . . . that was a very loving act.

P: (Cries, sobs.) (Long pause.)

T: It was love for your unborn child. In a sense, you didn't want to pass the abuse down to the next generation.[8]

---

8. Mary Main remarked that she felt the patient harbored the unconscious fear of being killed by her child (if ever conceived).

(Dr. Neborsky connects the intergenerational abuse to the patient's self-abuse.)

T: I hope that if anything happens out of this interview, that you're real clear on self-abuse and what is self-abuse.

P: Yeah, I think I know (nods).

T: You're not rationalizing it or intellectualizing it? Not shaming yourself, of course.

P: No, observing it.

T: Yeah, and remember the truth. Do you want to treat yourself the way your grandmother treated you? Do you want to treat yourself the way your mother treated you? Do you want to do that?

P: No.

T: See, call a spade a spade, OK? How would you like me to be of assistance? Is there anything you want from me here in your future? Is there anything you want me to do?

P: I don't know. Um . . . I think, really that I might want to come back.

T: OK.

P: (Long pause) I think I want to look more at the issue . . . have an autonomy without being self-destructive.

T: OK.

P: That's all that's coming up right now.

T: That's huge! (Both laugh.)

The patient showed a remarkable response to the six-hour therapy. She rededicated herself to her health, diet and exercise program. Her self esteem improved, depression and anxiety lifted, and her relationship with her husband became more loving and intimate.

Conclusion

Mary Main has already described in an earlier chapter how trauma is transmitted from parent to child. But Mary has also left us with the incredibly optimistic notion that insecurely attached infants can be changed through life's experience. Psychotherapy can be categorized as a life experience. My role in this chapter is to begin to suggest ways to facilitate that process.

I want to underscore what Allan Schore mentioned at the end of his presentation. Allan stated that any serious remedial therapy must be directed toward the unconscious. This book offers compelling evidence that the disturbances in affect regulation are largely right hemisphere or lower brain stem phenomena. They are by definition non-verbal. As Bessel Van Der Kolk correctly pointed out many verbally based talk therapies are destined to fail because they are ineffective in restoring normative affect regulation. Therefore, we must learn to use non-interpretive therapeutic approaches to help our patients move from insecure states to earned secure states. Dan Segal has shared with us the brain's desire to avoid change by maintaining a balance between chaos and rigidity. The task of the dynamic therapist is to create a shift in the brain systems so that a new equilibrium develops that is more flexible, more adaptive, and free of stress.

The method that I have presented was learned under a mentorship with Habib Davanloo of McGill University. From him I learned systematic techniques to gain rapid access to unconscious affects in the initial therapeutic contact with patients. What I have done is merge this technique with the recent discoveries of attachment theory and self-regulation. Through the use of these non-interpretive techniques, access to dissociated feeling states can be rapidly experienced, processed, and integrated. These methodologies along with EMDR are the two most powerful therapies that I've witnessed that can bring about *both* rapid and long lasting change.

All of the authors of this book share a common interest. We are interested in the process of change. No matter what our orientation, we are in the business of helping people change the way they feel, the way they behave, or the way they think. Over my career I've had the privilege of interacting with some great minds that have dedicated themselves to addressing the *most efficient* ways to accomplish that task. Some of those very best minds are represented in this volume.

Now, in truth, the applied science of psychotherapy is a remarkably young science. Psychotherapy itself is only 150 years old. The application of the scientific method to the process of psychotherapy is perhaps only seventy-five years old. The purpose of my chapter is to highlight the application of fifty years of intensive research in the process of psychotherapy to the clinical situation. I want to suggest that dynamic psychotherapy holds enormous untapped potential to help our patients change in dramatic ways that may be underestimated by large sectors of the professional community.

The backbone of short-term dynamic treatment is the clinician's ability to recognize the patient's dilemma. The patients come for treatment because they are suffering and want help, but they are truly unable, as Bessel pointed out, to do what is required to overcome their difficulties. What is required of them is to *feel* the emotions in the therapeutic dyad, which were not safe for them to feel at an earlier time and an earlier place. They have learned to defend against these experiences and are hence locked in a painful place from which there seems to be no escape. Their inability to feel despite their willingness to do so, is called resistance.

Now I want to return to Mary Main's wonderful image of Charles Darwin throwing the tortoise into the ocean and him swimming back to home base. The instinctual force in that turtle exists in all of us. That force is attachment. Davanloo recognized that the therapist could use that force itself, as a tool to get these patient's to feel. He called that tool the unconscious therapeutic alliance. You see, the patient wants to receive help, they want care; they want closeness, comfort, and connection. The therapist needs to communicate to the patient that they can have it, *but to do so they have to swim to shore.* They have to overcome the resistance that sits between you and them. You have to make it clear to them that that's their responsibility, that you're not going to magically and omnipotently do it for them. No, they're going to have to do it themselves. Naturally, they are going to become anxious because they're in a conflict. The patient wants to maintain their resistance, *but they also want to get to shore.* This creates an approach/avoidance conflict and then the therapy starts. Or better stated, we're into "the unconscious space." Entry into "the unconscious space" allows for the resolution of either hypo arousal states wherein all emotion is shut down, or hyper arousal states where the patient is agitated or anxious from affect flooding. The curative factor, different from EMDR is attachment-based where the patient experiences *containment* of the affect through the interpersonal presence of the therapist. Containment, mirroring, and attunement are remarkably soothing to adults as well as children. The crucial variable is lowering the anxiety enough so that the patient can contact the core emotional state, that heretofore frightened them. This covers point one of healing trauma outlined in the introduction. What about the second point, putting trauma into a spiritual/philosophical continuum? Patients undergoing this therapy occasionally compare it to the *transcendent* religious experiences. Frequently they discover a continuous panoramic vision of life, and see that the trauma they have suffered has in some fashion, given them the opportunity to explore places in themselves that would have otherwise been locked shut. They report that their brains are opened up to new realities and ways of experiencing themselves, their emotions and others. They report the fact that they are more tuned in to their loving, empathic capacity than before the trauma. This, in and of itself, gives some meaning to their suffering.

In closing, before affect regulation theory our clinical predecessors relied on less sophisticated models to understand and explore the unconscious. Today we have the clinical tools to repair deeply embedded and disrupted neural networks. We are living in an age in which an interpersonal neurobiology is becoming a reality. It's an exciting time for the practice of psychotherapy.

BIBLIOGRAPHY

Ainsworth, M. D. S., Blehar, M. C., Waters, E., & Wall, S. (1978). *Patterns of attachment: A psychological study of the Strange Situation.* Hillsdale, NJ: Erlbaum.

Ainsworth, M. D. S. & Eichberg, C. (1991). Effects on infant-mother attachment of mother's unresolved loss of an attachment figure, or other traumatic experience. In C. M. Parkes, J. Stevenson-Hinde, & P. Marris (Eds.), *Attachment across the life cycle* (pp. 160–186). London: Routledge.

Bowlby, J. (1969). *Attachment and loss: Vol. 1. Attachment.* New York: Basic Books.

Bowlby, J. (1973). *Attachment and loss: Vol. 2. Separation and anger.* New York: Basic Books.

Bowlby, J. (1980). *Attachment and loss: Vol. 3. Loss: Sadness and depression.* New York: Basic Books.

Bowlby, J. (1988). *A secure base: Parent-child attachment and healthy human development.* New York: Basic Books.

Davanloo, H. (1988a). Clinical manifestations of superego pathology. Part II. The resistance of the superego and the liberation of the paralyzed ego. *International Journal of Short-Term Psychotherapy, 3,* 1–24.

Davanloo, H. (1988b). The technique of unlocking the unconscious. Part II. Partial unlocking of the unconscious. *International Journal of Short-Term Psychotherapy, 3 (2),* 123–159.

Davanloo, H. (1988b). The technique of unlocking of the unconscious. Part I. *International Journal of Short-Term Psychotherapy, 3 (2),* 99–121.

Davanloo, H. (1988c). The technique of unlocking of the unconscious. Part II. Partial unlocking of the unconscious. *International Journal of Short-Term Psychotherapy, 3 (2),* 123–159.

Davanloo, H. (1989a). Central dynamic sequence in the unlocking of the unconscious and comprehensive trial therapy. Part I. Major unlocking. *International Journal of Short-Term Psychotherapy, 4 (1),* 1–33.

Davanloo, H. (1989b). Central dynamic sequence in the major unlocking of the unconscious and comprehensive trial therapy. Part II. The course of trial therapy after the initial breakthrough. *International Journal of Short-Term Psychotherapy, 4 (1),* 35–66.

Davanloo, H. (1989c). The technique of unlocking the unconscious in patients suffering from functional disorder. Part I. Restructuring ego's defenses. *International Journal of Short-Term Psychotherapy, 4 (2),* 93–116.

Davanloo, H. (1989d). The technique of unlocking the unconscious in patients suffering from functional disorders. Part II. Direct view of the dynamic unconscious. *International Journal of Short-Term Psychotherapy, 4 (2),* 117–148.

Davanloo, H. (1990). *Unlocking the Unconscious.* Chichester: Wiley.

Davanloo, H. (1995a). Intensive short-term dynamic psychotherapy: spectrum of psycho-neurotic disorders. *International Journal of Short-Term Psychotherapy, 10 (3, 4),* 121–155.

Davanloo, H. (1995b). Intensive short-term dynamic psychotherapy: technique of partial and major unlocking of the unconscious with a highly resistant patient. Part I. Partial unlocking of the unconscious. *International Journal of Short-Term Psychotherapy, 10 (3, 4),* 157–181.

Davanloo, H. (1995c). Intensive short-term dynamic psychotherapy: major unlocking of the unconscious. Part II. The course of the trial therapy after partial unlocking. *International Journal of Short-Term Psychotherapy, 10 (3, 4),* 183–230.

Davanloo, H. (1996a). Management of tactical defenses in intensive short-term dynamic psychotherapy. Part I. Overview, tactical defenses of cover words and indirect speech. *International Journal of Short-Term Psychotherapy, 11 (3),* 129–152.

Davanloo, H. (1996b). Management of tactical defenses in intensive short-term dynamic psychotherapy. Part II. Spectrum of tactical defenses. *International Journal of Short-Term Psychotherapy, 11 (3),* 153–199.

Davanloo, H. (1999). Intensive short-term dynamic psychotherapy—central dynamic sequence: Phase of pressure. *International Journal of Short-Term Psychotherapy, 13:4,* 211–233.

Davanloo, H. (1999). Intensive short-term dynamic psychotherapy—central dynamic sequence: Phase of challenge. *International Journal of Short-Term Psychotherapy, 13:4,* 237–260.

Davanloo, H. (1999). Intensive short-term dynamic psychotherapy—central dynamic sequence: Head-on collision with resistance. *International Journal of Short-Term Psychotherapy, 13:4,* 263–280.

Emde, R. (1983). The prerepresentational self and its affective core. *The Psychoanalytic Study of the Child,* 38:165–192. New haven, CT: Yale University Press.

Erikson, E. H. (1963). *Childhood and society.* 2nd ed. New York: W. W. Norton & Company.

Fonagy, P, Gergely, G., Jurist, E.L, and Target, M. (2002) Affect Regulation, Mentalization, and the Development of the Self. New York: Other Press.

Freud, A. (1967). Comment on trauma. In: *Psychic Trauma,* ed. S.S. Furst. New York: Basic Books, pp. 235–245.0

Freud, S. (1911). *Remembering, Repeating, and Working Through. Standard Edition,* 12:150. London: Hogarth Press, 1959.

Freud, S. (1918). *Introduction to Psychoanalysis and the War Neurosis. Standard Edition,* 17:207–210. London: Hogarth Press, 1959.

Freud, S. (1926). *Inhibitions, Symptoms, and Anxiety. Standard Edition,* 20:75–175. London: Hogarth Press, 1959.

Jones, J.M. (1995). *Affects as process.* Hillsdale, New Jersey: Analytic Press.

Korn, Martin (2001)

Kahn, M (1963). The concept of cumulative trauma. *The Psychoanalytic Study of the Child,.* New haven, CT: Yale University Press.

Main, M. (1991). Metacognitive knowledge, metacognitive monitoring, and singular (coherent) versus multiple (incoherent) models of attachment: Findings and directions for future research. In C. M. Parkes, J. Stenson-Hinde, & P. Marris (Eds.), *Attachment across the life cycle* (pp. 127–159). London: Routledge.

Main, M. (1993). Discourse, prediction, and recent studies in attachment: Implications for psychoanalysis. *Journal of the American Psychoanalytic Association, 41,* 209–244.

Main, M. (1995). Attachment: Overview, with implications for clinical work. In S. Goldberg, R. Muir, & J. Kerr (Eds.), *Attachment theory: Social, developmental and clinical perspectives* (pp. 407–474). Hillsdale, NJ: Analytic Press.

Main, M. (1996). Introduction to the special section on attachment and psychopathology: 2. Overview of the field of attachment. *Journal of Consulting and Clinical Psychology, 64,* 237–243.

Main, M. (in press). The Adult Attachment Interview: Fear, attention, safety and discourse processes. *Journal of the American Psychoanalytic Association.*

Main, M. & Goldwyn, R. (1984). *Adult attachment scoring and classification system.* Unpublished manuscript, University of California at Berkeley.

Main, M. & Goldwyn, R. (1998). *Adult attachment scoring and classification systems* (Version 6.3). Unpublished manuscript, University of California at Berkeley.

Main, M. & Hesse, E. (1990). Parent's unresolved traumatic experiences are related to infant disorganized status: Is frightened and/or frightening parental behavior the linking mechanism? In M. T. Greenberg, D. Cicchetti, & E. M. Cummings (Eds.), *Attachment in the preschool years: Theory, research, and intervention* (pp. 161–182). Chicago: University of Chicago Press.

Main, M., Kaplan, N., & Cassidy, J. (1985). Security in infancy, childhood, and adulthood: A move to the level of representation. In I. Bretherton & E. Waters (Eds.), Growing points of attachment theory and research. *Monographs of the Society for Research in Child Development, 50* (2–3 Serial No. 209), 66–104.

Main, M. & Morgan, H. (1996). Disorganization and disorientation in infant Strange Situation behavior: Phenotypic resemblance to dissociative states. In L. K. Michelson & W. J. Ray (Eds.), *Handbook of dissociation: Theoretical, empirical, and clinical perspectives* (pp. 121–160). Chicago: University of Chicago Press.

Main, M. & Solomon, J. (1986). Discovery of an insecure-disorganized/disoriented attachment pattern. In T. B. Brazelton & M. Yogman (Eds.), *Affective development in infancy* (pp. 95–124). Norwood, NJ: Ablex.

Main, M. & Solomon, J. (1990). Procedures for identifying infants as disorganized/disoriented during the Ainsworth Strange Situation. In M. T. Greenberg, D. Cicchetti, & E. M. Cummings (Eds.), *Attachment in the preschool years: Theory, research, and intervention* (pp. 121–160). Chicago: University of Chicago Press.

Neborsky, R.J. (1998) A new metapsychology of the unconscious. UCSD Cutting Edge Conference. *Short-Term Therapy for Long-Term Change.* La Jolla, California.

Neborsky, R.J. (2000) A study in hysteria. One-day symposium. Lifespan Learning Institute. November 2, Los Angeles, California.

Neborsky, R.J., Janowsky, D (1980) Hypothesized common mechanisms in the psychopharmacologic and psychotherapeutic treatment of depression. *Psychiatric Annals*

Schore, A. N. (1996). The experience-dependent maturation of a regulatory system in the orbital prefrontal cortex and the origin of developmental psychopathology. *Development and Psychopathology, 8,* 59–87.

Schore, A. N. (1997). Early organization of the nonlinear right brain and development of a predisposition to psychiatric disorders. *Development and Psychopathology, 9,* 595–631.

Schore, A. N. (1998). The experience-dependent maturation of an evaluative system in the cortex. In K. H. Pribram & J. King (Eds.), *Brain and values: Is a biological science of values possible?* (pp. 337–358). Mahway, NJ: Erlbaum.

Schore, A. N. (in press). Clinical Implications of a neurobiological model of projective identification. In S. Alhanti, Ed *Primitive Mental States, Volume III "Pre- and Peri-natal influences on personality development."* ESF Publishers.

Shapiro, F. (1995) *Eye Movement Desensitization and Reprocessing : Basic Principles, Protocols and Procedures.* New York: Guilford.

Siegel, D. J. (1995). Memory, trauma, and psychotherapy: A cognitive science view. *Journal of Psychotherapy Practice and Research, 4,* 93–122.

Siegel, D. J. (1999). *The developing mind.* New York: Guilford Press.

Solomon, M.F., Neborsky, R. J., McCullough, L., Alpert, M., Shapiro, F., Malan, D.M., (2001 in press) *Short-Term Therapy for Long-Term Change.* New York: W.W. Norton and Co.

Stern, D. N. (1985). *The interpersonal world of the infant.* New York: Basic Books.

Stroufe, L.A., Egeland, B., & Krentger, T. (1990). The fate of early experience following developmental change: Longitudinal approaches to individual adaptation in childhood. *Child Development,* 54, 1615–1627.

Van der Kolk, B. (1989). The compulsion to repeat the trauma. *Psychiatric Clinics of North America, 1.*

"A Clinical Model for the Comprehensive Treatment of Trauma Using an Affect Experiencing-Attachment Theory Approach" in Solomon, M. & Siegel, D., *Healing Trauma.* New York. WW. Norton & Company, 2003. The author also wishes to thank WW. Norton & Co. for their permission to reproduce parts of Chapter 7 "Attachment Bonds and Intimacy: Can the Primary Imprint of Love Change?" by Robert J. Neborsky and Marion F. Solomon in *Short-Term Therapy for Long-Term Change.*

Shame and Guilt from a Developmental Neuroscience Perspective

Implications for Technique in Intensive Short-Term Dynamic Psychotherapy

The role of shame in patient pathology and ISTDP's metapsychology has been largely ignored. The author of the following article posits that understanding the role of shame, and differentiating it from guilt, is of critical importance in identifying and healing emotional trauma in highly resistant patients. The author discusses the neurobiological basis of shame, its psychological and social functions, and its course of development in the mother-child dyad. The author goes on the suggest that only when shame is recognized and effectively dealt with post-breakthrough can the therapist assume the affect-containment mirroring function that early caregivers failed at, and thus ensure a patient's freedom from symptoms.

Introduction

The therapeutic cornerstone of intensive short-term dynamic psychotherapy is the bringing of relationally based unconscious affect into consciousness. Following completion of that task, the patient and therapist collaborate to resolve the pathogenic power of the affects. Davanloo (1988, 89, 95) and others have written extensively about making anxiety conscious, along with sadness-grief, rage, and guilt. A review of the literature on intensive short-term dynamic psychotherapy shows remarkably little writing on shame and no mention of new findings from affective neuroscience. The metapsychology of intensive short-term dynamic psychotherapy, as described by Davanloo (1988a), is a guilt-based system of psychopathology, and there is no mention of the pathogenic nature of shame. In this article, I will address that omission.

Origins, Definitions, and Functions of Shame and Guilt

Etymologically, shame means, "to cover." This is an apt psychological definition as well. Child developmentalists (Broucek, 1982), (Stern, 1985), (Kaufman, 1989) view the affect of shame as an *inhibitory* affect that seems to become available to infants by around 18 months of life. By an inhibitory affect, they mean that shame changes infants from hyper-aroused states to hypo-aroused states. Neurobiological research reveals shame to originate from activation of the parasympathetic nervous system. Specifically, the shame system originates in the dorsal medial nucleus of the hypothalamus (Schore, 1998). Activation of this area causes changes in mood, endocrine function, and involuntary (smooth) muscle activity.

From infant observation, Tompkins (1962) sees shame originating in the mother-infant dyad as a self-protective reaction when attunement disruptions occur. Schore also points out that in mother-infant dysregulated dyads shame protects the infant from neurological trauma from over-excitation following attachment failure. We now know that in infancy until the third year of life, the right hemisphere is the dominant hemisphere. So, it seems likely that shame is a predominately right hemisphere emotion with little need for left hemisphere participation. As development proceeds, shame begins to differentiate itself away from dyadic origins as an arousal regulator, and eventually becomes part of a self-regulatory apparatus for social behavior.

The role of shame in psychological functioning is complex and multi-tiered. Eventually, it develops a signal role like fear. One role of shame is to give the self immediate assessment about actual or potential social boundary violations. Additionally, in a very simple way, shame gives feedback to the self as to perceived social rank as well as an ultimate measure of one's value or worth within a group. Each individual develops an unconscious "set point" by which they measure their actual self from their ideal self. This largely unconscious system determines whether the self is full of self-esteem or, conversely, shame.

Self-esteem correlates with pride. The pre-verbal roots of pride lie in attunement experiences wherein co-regulation of affect in the mother-infant dyad is successful and rather than a "covering" response the action tendency is *to exhibit* oneself as a source of joy and pleasure.

Once shame is established as a signal affect in the child's psyche, it may become a tool, which can be activated by parental disapproval—negative judgment—and it can be activated by a word, a look, a tone of voice, or a sentence. Conversely, shame-states can be transmitted from child to parent when the child disapproves of the parental actions. The activation of signal shame frequently activates anger toward the shaming source when one's sense of self is threatened by the negative judgment. This transaction is seen frequently in narcissistic parents. This is a very intricate intrapsychic and interpersonal process which will be elaborated upon in future papers.

Since the time of Freud (1913, 1926), guilt has been seen as an inhibitory affect as well. The capacity for guilt is seen to come on later in child development than it does for shame. I believe guilt may actually evolve or differentiate itself from the same neuronal matrix of the shame system that is rapidly shaping itself based on earlier developmental interaction with caregivers. In Freudian models and child developmental observation, guilt appears between ages three to six, coincident with the neurological development and domination of the left hemisphere. So the fibers of the guilt system are more thoroughly distributed throughout the brain than the shame system and require transmission of information across the Corpus Callosum (Schore, personal communication). Shame, like attunement failure rage, is a largely right brain (Amygdala) phenomenon. So when the child develops the capacity for self-observation, and story making about oneself, as well as a concept of social norms, guilt emerges as an affect. Darwin (1814) and Bowlby (1980) both have emphasized the importance of identifying the *action tendency* to biologically programmed emotion. The action tendency of guilt is seeking punishment. Much like shame, guilt has social evolutionary value. Freud (1913) addressed this issue in *Totem and Taboo.* Guilt adaptively controls the upsurge of sexually driven aggression and competition between males for female sexual attention and satisfaction as well as protecting the species from genetic degradation by incest. Sons don't usually kill their fathers to consummate incest with mothers; fathers don't usually abandon their wives for their daughters; mothers don't usually consummate incest with their sons; nor do they usually kill their children when food supplies are scant. Historically, the punishment for the violation of these social barriers has been severe. When the French revolutionary council accused Marie Antoinette, the charge against her was incest with her six-year-old son as well as treason. Treason was the more difficult charge to prove so she was vigorously prosecuted for incest. Her son was separated from her and forced by the prosecutors to testify against her. She refused to defend herself against these charges, was found guilty, and with this pretext, beheaded.

There is a confluence of these two emotions—shame and guilt—and the same triggers that stimulate shame can trigger guilt and both action tendencies are set off "to cover" and when repair is blocked to "seek punishment." This is frequently what we see in clinical practice. In prior writings I have described the "PASO" or primitive aggressive self organization (Neborsky, 2001). This is why I have placed shame and guilt on the same concentric circle, since they are both activated in complex transference feelings and at times are difficult to separate experientially. In 1987 Helen Bloch Lewis noted that shame is difficult to separate from guilt because one can trigger the other or both can be triggered by a single event. "They get into what I call a *tangle.* Shame gets into guilt and guilt gets into shame and whichever way, the person can't get out. In the forties when I was training, we called it a chronic state of guilt. It's guilt, too, but the role of shame in the whole mess has been underestimated."

Davanloo's Approach: Semantic and Developmental Confusion

Davanloo's theories were developed through careful clinical observation and systematic analysis of adult patients. So Davanloo's theories are a top down pragmatic approach, much like Freud's was with psychoanalysis. Even though this approach has its merits, it also has its limitations since it ignores research from other areas which may have different conclusions. The field of intensive short-term dynamic psychotherapy will only grow and prosper as a discipline if it is open ended, and welcomes research that can increase the power and effectiveness of an already potent treatment.

Studying Davanloo's (1989) ideas show that his system of pathology is primarily a guilt based system. He sees that mental health is a function of sustained attachment bonds between caregiver and child across time. The longer these healthy bonds are sustained, the lower resistance these patient's will be (left side of the spectrum); the more disturbed these bonds are or the earlier in development they have been broken, then the more resistant and severe the psychopathology will be, all the way to fragile, narcissistic and borderline states (right side of spectrum).

Davanloo's scheme of psychopathology for moderate to high resistant cases sees the cascade of emotions being triggered by loss of the "good enough" (Winnicott, 1960) caregiver. Davanloo labels the first experience as pain of trauma that is converted into rage against the caregiver. The caregiver is "destroyed" by the child's rage and the corpse of the caregiver is internalized as guilt and symptom. The unconscious rage and other feelings are defended against (repressed) in childhood and lie dormant to be re-activated in adult life. Patient after patient (thousands by now) validate his observations when they look into the eyes of the murdered body of the therapist and see the eyes of the offending caregiver and feel grief and guilt and then their unconscious tells us the story of their developmental trauma.

If we analyze the breakthrough carefully, we can observe the following hypothesized neurobiological phenomena. Asking the patient to look (most likely) activates the right hemisphere occipital cortex and associated hippocampal memory tracts. The patient looks at the corpse of someone they were attached to and once loved. This stimulates guilt—the left hemisphere emotion—in non-psychopathic people. Guilt is about transgression and wrongful acts, but what has created the unconscious murderous rage? The rage was created by broken or lost attachment bond. Davanloo's research shows that patients on the left (healthy side) of the spectrum have had the attachment bonds broken later in their development—frequently post six years of age.

The clinical genius of Davanloo is confirmed by the fact that he recognized this intuitively and called it "pain of trauma." At a conference hosted by the now-defunct San Diego Institute (Neborsky, 1984), Davanloo asked the rhetorical question: "in the structural model where is pain?" It has taken me literally 26 years to understand the answer to that question.

Reformulation of Psychopathology and Intensive Short-Term Dynamic Psychotherapy Technique from Modern Neurobiology Research

The rage of covert attachment trauma before age three is a more complicated clinical problem. These patients, who frequently fit into the fragile category, are more difficult to treat. Their unconscious rage is more primitive, their symptoms more diffuse, and relationships more disturbed. They also have a higher incidence of psycho-physiologic disorders (parasympathetically mediated).

If what Schore reports is true, and the capacity to experience guilt is not neurologically available until around three, we are dealing with non-verbal dyadic attunement traumas in these patients. This disputes the Kleinian model of pre-Oedipal guilt which seems so seductive when looking at our clinical data (Klein, 1926). I believe what we frequently observe with this category of patient is the co-mingling of two affect regulating systems that activated by the process of intensive short-term dynamic psychotherapy. One is the rage-shame system and the other is the rage-guilt system.

What I believe we are actually seeing is the activation of two distinct brain systems which develop at different times. The attachment system, the most primitive system, is activated by the transference, and because it was historically disrupted, it carries with it severe anger, dysregulation, and shame interruption circuits as well as the rage-guilt (DNA based, *i.e.,* genetic prohibition) over destruction of biologic relative system which came on line coincident with ages three to six.

The transformative power of the breakthrough is that we actively separate these co-mingled systems and remove guilt from the attachment system, and thus make repair of the damaged attachment system possible. Frequently in my practice after the breakthrough of the rage, grief, and guilt has passed, a rising feeling emerges that is shut down, and this requires intervention. This I believe is emerging shame to shut off the traumatic feeling that the patient unconsciously anticipates will be rejected, ignored, or over-activated by the therapist (like it once was by the caregiver). These traumatic feelings are the very ones in which failed attunement occurred in the non-verbal past. If the therapist intervenes successfully, the patient's memory system opens and repressed memories of relational failure-events emerge with sharp here-and-now flashback form. The therapeutic process moves forward and effects more and more separation and differentiation of these separate systems. The working through in intensive short-term dynamic psychotherapy eventually shifts to sadness and grief about the covert losses in the patient's life, and the rage-shame extinguishes. The therapist takes over the affect containment mirroring function for the patient that the offending caregiver was not able to supply. In so doing the patient becomes free of symptoms, more zestful and capable of joyful relational activity. Termination occurs when separation of these different systems is complete and normalized.

For those who are unfamiliar with the attachment system, it was first described by Bowlby (1969) in England. It is in all mammals and even present in some sub-mammals in one form or another. Basically, attachment is the biologically programmed relationship between mother infant pair bonds in which the infant specifically recognizes the mother separate from others and maintains proximity to her. On the next level, attachment is the specific behavior of the mother that creates comfort for the infant when the infant shows signs of distress. These interactions occur over time and create specific patterns of handling emotion in the mother-infant dyad. Specific types of reactions of mothers determine whether the child becomes secure or insecure in their attachment style. By far and away the greatest determinant of insecure attachment is unresolved trauma in the life history of the infant's mother. This is greater than temperament or sensitivity by high degrees of statistical significance.

Therefore, I have come to believe that the therapist's capacity for attunement to genuine emotion is a critical factor for the success of intensive short-term dynamic psychotherapy. The therapist's ability to affectively contain, mirror, or empathically resonate to rage, sadness, and grief, and to undo the shame and/or guilt co-mingled with these emotions, maybe the single most important curative factor in the therapy. While the negative consequences of poor training are self-evident, I would like to add that unresolved trauma in the intensive short-term dynamic psychotherapist will almost certainly interfere with successful repair of the patient's attachment system, and thus may well result in the treatments.

Narcissism, Shame, Neglect and Abuse

Many of our patients suffer from narcissism (empathic lack, self-aggrandizement) that is the result of the pain of trauma inflicted by narcissistic parents. Each of these parent-child dyads suffer from inter-generational transmission of trauma on the basis of attachment failure (Neborsky, 2002). Contrary to many theories of narcissism, it is my thesis that narcissistic patients do not suffer from excessive shame, but an *inability* to tolerate shame states at all. These people are exquisitely sensitive to loss of attunement in relationships and go into rage, dysregulation, shame cycles at the drop of a hat. They then develop complex compensatory strategies to protect themselves from relational trauma. They become excessively controlling, arrogant, powerful, dismissive, distant, and/or withholding to avoid the closeness and complex feelings of past trauma re-activated in intimate relationships. Part of their repertoire can be aggressive attacking sadism that reduces their partners to dysregulated buckets of rage-shame and rage-guilt (like they once were treated in relationships).

Children of parents with narcissistic difficulties become hyper-attuned to the psychological triggers of their caregivers and report "walking on egg shells" or exhibit role reversing comfort behaviors to attempt to stabilize the parent's volatile emotions. Other narcissistic parents turn cold when the child's emotional needs activate their trauma, and the rage-shame trauma is transmitted to the child in that way. These children frequently become dismissive bullies who control and push others away or masochistic doormats who are victims of their loved ones. Adults and parents who molest children frequently fall into one of the above categories. The adult cannot tolerate the complex feelings in adult intimate relationships because of the constant threat of activating trauma, so they act out the fantasy of trauma free love with a child over whom they have control. The sexual act becomes a role reversal wherein they (the caregiver) in fantasy give the child the loving experience they longed for as a child. Their psychotic fantasy is that of receiving from their parent complete attunement to their physical/emotional selves. In reality, the psychopathic transaction in fact recreates the trauma and dysregulates the child, creating a psychoneurosis.

Confusing Ways Shame Presents in the Clinical Setting: Defense *and/or* Feeling

Figure 1 shows the traditional triangle of conflict modified to include the rage-shame cycle. Clinically, shame is frequently used defensively, before a patient is unlocked. It can be used tactically to cover deeper feelings; it can be used as a resistance against emotional closeness; or it can become part of the superego as a way of punishing the self.

Figure 1. Reconceived Triangle of Conflict Paradigm for Patient with Attunement Trauma

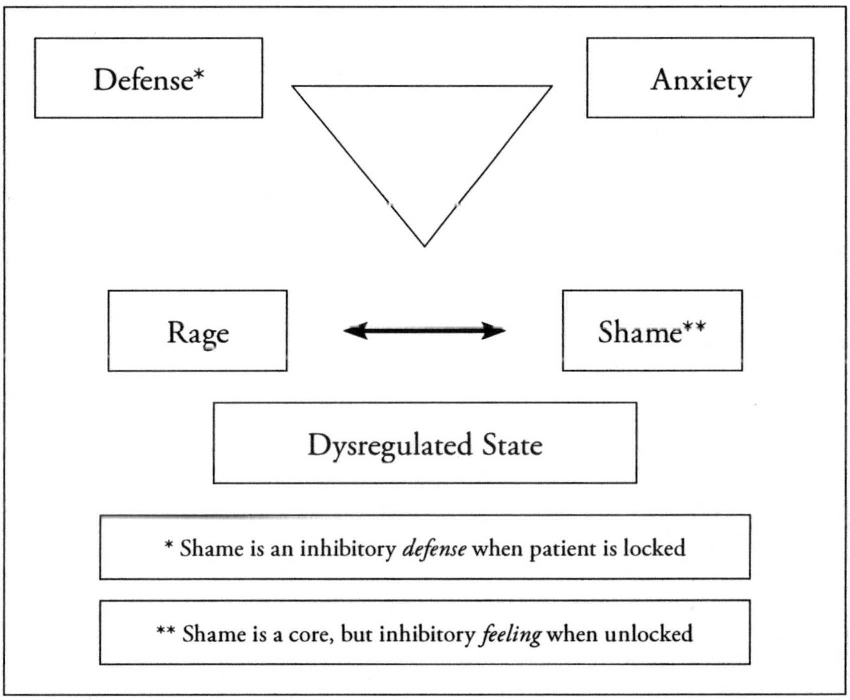

This is a diagram which shows the tradition triangle of conflict modified to include the rage-shame cycle that was heretofore called "pain of trauma." Clinicians are frequently confused by the defensive affect of shame before breakthrough, which becomes a core affect after the guilt is experienced and relieved.

In the cases I am describing, this phenomenon occurs after resistance and unconscious anxiety has been defeated by the therapeutic alliance and when the patient is fully in touch with their murderous feeling with clear visualization of their behavior, and they begin to "shut down." There is no noticeable anxiety about the impulse. There is simply a subtle shutting off of the feeling, which needs intervention or "re-ignition" (attunement to the shut down) by the therapist. I would be interested to hear if other colleagues have noticed this phenomenon as well. What follows is a clinical example of this phenomenon in the form of an edited transcript of a videotape presented at the Natura Artis Magistra Conference, Amsterdam, Netherlands September 2002.

Case Presentation: Primal Fear When a Parent turns Predator

This patient presented for intensive short-term dynamic psychotherapy following unsuccessful intensive short-term dynamic psychotherapy treatment with another practitioner also trained by Davanloo but without my focus on shame. She is a thirty-two-year old healthcare practitioner, married, mother of one daughter age 3. Her difficulties were anger outbursts, anxiety, and depression along with unresolved relational issues with her parents and in-laws. She reported no parenting difficulties. As the interview unfolded she reported sexual molestation by her father during age 6–9 with concurrent untreated or noticed childhood depression. (The father later confirmed this history in a telephone conversation to me: He said he did molest her and now feels sorry. He declined the suggestion of therapy as he did not trust that a psychotherapist would help him figure out why he became a perpetrator.

Transcript

Initial Session, August 2001

The therapist begins this initial session by asking the patient to describe her areas of disturbance.

P: Mmm . . . well, a couple of things . . . I think a big thing for me is that I have a problem with . . . um . . . intimacy or with . . . developing closeness with people. I've always had that problem and . . . that's something I would like to address.

T: Uh huh.

P: And I um . . . have a problem with . . . just emotion in general. I think I'm, I'm, um . . . unable to feel many emotions and, and then at times things seem to come to a head for me and I'll explode with anger, um . . . and the other emotion that I, that I experience a lot is um . . . sadness. But I have a really hard time . . . you know, expressing or knowing what I'm feeling. I'm not able to really . . . I don't feel a thing, I know there's something going on but I don't know what it is a lot of times.

T: Uh huh. Uh huh.

P: Um . . . so I have . . .

T: So it's kind of a wall between you and the feeling. You know the feeling's there but it's hard to put your finger on it.

P: Uh huh. Exactly. Unless it's anger, and that can come out in pretty ugly ways and I guess that would be my main concern is, um . . . that sometimes it just comes out and I don't . . . I don't want to be that ugly, angry person.

T: Give me an example of what you mean.

P: Um . . . yesterday speaking on the phone with the operator, I'm getting angry with her 'cause she can't find the number I need, and then having a verbal altercation with the operator.

T: Uh huh. And I'm not sure how that's not under control. That's the point I'm trying to understand.

P: Uh . . . it just seems like . . . I think it's not under my control because I wouldn't choose to act that way towards someone, if I could, you know, choose how I wanted to behave . . . I wouldn't behave in that way. And it just seems like . . . something is triggered in me, it's like a little button is pushed or knob is turned and . . . it's almost like another person.

T: Well, what happened, exactly, I mean, what was the . . . Did you notice inside, in this process of change from, you know, the way you are perhaps now to the way you were then. What did you note inside? What was your awareness?

P: Um . . . I feel like, kind of like pressure inside . . .

T: Uh huh.

P: And . . . like something wants to explode.

T: Uh huh. And does it happen just like that, or is there a good, you know, I mean, is there a slope to it? Does the anger gradually build?

P: I think it's more . . . it's more, um . . . just very fast and immediate.

T: More of a strike.

P: Yeah.

T: Up, and huge pressure.

P: I . . . I believe so. It's hard . . . like I said . . . I feel that I'm kind of out of touch with how I feel.

T: Wow.

P: And so I can't . . .

T: Well, what do you make of that? I mean . . .

P: I'm just disconnecting from my feelings.

T: Yeah.

P: They're dangerous. But, you know, in my subconscious, I've prevented myself from feeling ever since I was a little kid because . . . it was too dangerous to deal with all of those feelings and um . . . I had to prevent myself from feeling them because they were just too dangerous. I was a little kid and I couldn't have the anger to a point where I was feeling it. It was self-preservation basically. You know, that was my way of coping with it. It's what everyone does.

T: Well . . . that makes a lot of sense to me.

P: Uh huh.

T: You know . . . I mean . . .

P: Yeah. It worked then, but it's not . . . it's not functioning now.

T: Uh huh. Uh huh. Now, it was so noticeable that you said it was "dangerous." That those words came out of you, you know. Was there any emotion consistent with danger? 'Cause there obviously was that thought, I mean, "It's dangerous."

P: I just said it now?

T: Uh huh.

P: I don't know. I feel very sad.

T: Yeah, you do. Yeah. No question about that.

P: Hmmm . . . well, I'm not sure.

T: Well, let's talk about sadness for a moment.

P: OK.

T: What comes into your mind about your sadness?

P: I just have a lot of pain and . . . and . . . feeling of um . . . loss . . . and feeling of . . . just greatly missed um . . . potential, um . . . missed opportunities . . . and greatly missed um . . . relationships, and . . . it's just a big loss.

T: And, the cause of that, you follow me? The cause of that loss is what? What was the . . . ?

P: Um . . . I was abandoned, basically, by my parents. I knew they were there, but you know, they were not there for me. Um . . . my parents were . . . just both . . . abusive, and I think I had to um . . . just take care of myself. Not physically, but emotionally, and I've been alone since I was a little kid.

T: That's a lot to be sad about.

P: Hmm.

T: Tremendous amount to be sad about, isn't it?

P: Yeah.

T: Hmm huh. Now, I would also say that, you know, our ability to do much about those losses . . . it's fairly limited, I mean . . .

P: Uh, huh.

T: That in the past that has been . . . been lost, truly can't be recovered, I mean it's . . .

P: That's true.

T: So, our focus really ought to be on prevention of any future losses . . . any future . . .

P: Right.

T: . . . lost potential.

P: Right.

T: Now, I'm just going to bring to your attention what I was kind of looking for and what was missing . . . what I was kind of like . . . searching for. And, what I was searching for was a sense of fear, you know, when you said, "it's dangerous." I was looking for the emotion of fear, and I couldn't perceive it. I didn't see it in you at all.

P: Uh huh. Um . . . this is another issue for me . . . it's that I have a hard time distinguishing . . . because I . . . I have a hard time knowing what I'm feeling, then I have a hard time distinguishing what I'm actually feeling or what I've, you know, um . . . intellectualized that I should be feeling, or learned I should be feeling or experiencing.

T: Uh huh.

P: And so it's hard for me to distinguish, if I'm actually um . . . you know, the danger of expressing anger is dangerous because it was . . . it was dangerous as a child to express anger, my parents were . . .

T: But please, please bear with me. I love what you said . . . OK?

P: Uh huh.

T: Uh . . . that's fine, you know, you have trouble distinguishing this from that from this.

P: Uh huh.

T: Fair game, I mean, that's something I can really help you with.

P: Uh huh.

T: See, that's something we can really sink our teeth in . . .

P: Uh huh.

T: That can be learned . . .

P: OK.

T: Right? I mean that's what we would hope that we could accomplish.

P: Uh huh.

T: So I just want to make . . . idea. "It's dangerous" is an idea. It's a thought.

P: Right.

T: It's not a feeling.

P: Right.

T: OK. Keep this on an intellectual level, right?

P: Uh huh.

T: Then that kind of insures the outcome is going to be negative.

P: Uh huh.

T: See? So again . . . fear, or danger, OK . . . worry . . . is there an emotional part there, is there a feeling component . . . uh . . . to that?

P: I don't know how to get there . . . and how to . . .

T: So, the answer was: there isn't or there is? See, it's still . . .

P: I don't know.

T: Well, I don't understand how you can say you don't know.

P: I don't feel anything associated with it. But I'm thinking there should be!

T: Well, correct! OK, see . . . the honest answer is obviously the best answer, isn't it? The answer is . . .

P: No.

T: "No!"

P: Yeah, "no."

T: Yeah. So, you see, we've got something here that's so valuable to be able to approach. We can approach the, uh . . . the idea that you have this barrier against fear, OK? You can feel sadness. I saw it, I witnessed it. You can feel anger. We know from yesterday that you can feel anger, perhaps you even feel extreme anger, OK? And, you can even explain how anger feels. But when it comes to the emotion of fear, right? Then, for some reason, you've developed a way of extricating yourself from that part of feeling the experience.

P: Uh huh.

T: Does that make sense?

P: Yeah.

T: OK. So, it would be a very significant accomplishment if we could work on fear. It . . . do you have any memory or any recollection, um . . . a time where you knew you were afraid that you felt that emotion?

P: Um . . . I just remember standing in the hall . . . I don't know . . . I was a little kid and I had a nightmare and I wanted to go, you know, to my Mom . . . and I was afraid to go into my parents room and I was afraid to go back into my room. And I was, you know, standing afraid in the hall.

T: I see. And, what did you feel like? What do you remember?

P: All paralyzed. Then I couldn't move. I couldn't go back or forward.

T: Uh huh. Which is . . . in your memory again. Which is, again, very good and very crisp and very clear for obviously a painful event. But, you actually remember behavior, don't you? You remember motor paralysis.

P: Uh huh.

T: See, you're not remembering the experience of fear. Do you notice how that . . . ?

P: Yeah.

T: So, again I would say to you, or suggest to you that your defenses against the experience of fear are very, very strong! See. And one can appreciate that they perhaps had to be strong in order to maintain functioning.

P: Uh huh.

T: But in our work together, if you keep yourself defended against the experience of fear, my ability to offer you a therapeutic outcome is diminished.

P: Uh huh.

T: Until I know what it is that's frightening you, right? . . . we can't go into that process.

P: Uh huh.

T: Let's go back to here, OK? Where we were exploring the emotion of anger.

P: Uh huh.

T: OK? And you suggested that it was "dangerous."

P: Uh huh.

T: Anger itself was "dangerous." What did you have in mind?

P: Um . . . I think it's dangerous because it can cause me to act uh . . . outside of . . . out of control . . . outside of my control . . . to act in a dangerous way that's going to be harmful to me or other people. I'm afraid my anger is going to hurt someone . . . other people.

T: That's why I'm asking you to picture. How?

P: How it would hurt them?

T: Yeah.

P: By being . . . by causing pain to the emotional pain, by saying things that are painful.

T: Well, I hear what you're saying and of course on one level that's true. But, let's add now to what you're learning here. We've already learned that saying things that are hurtful, OK isn't a way of getting rid of the emotion of anger.

P: Uh huh. So, that's not real anger.

T: That's the defense.

P: I don't know. I'm having a hard time.

T: Again . . . I want to say these things to you 'cause I think it can clear up some misunderstandings, which to me is a really good response. The fact that you're having a hard time with this means that we're on all new territory for you. This is an approach which you haven't really, you know . . .

P: Uh huh.

T: . . . experienced before.

P: Right.

T: See? What's it just like for you sitting in the chair with me . . . when you're understanding that that attacking, verbal, lashing out behavior is defensive against experiencing the core angry part of the feeling? That that's actually a sabotaging defense . . . it gets rid of, it depressurizes, but it doesn't allow you to feel the core emotion. What's that like . . . when you just sit here and understand that?

P: Well, it's enlightening . . . um . . . and I never thought of it as separately, that was always . . . that was the anger, that is the anger, you know that . . .

T: Not the pressure-relief behavior?

P: I thought of it as the expression of anger.

T: Yeah.

P: So, you know, it's new . . . it's a new way of looking at it.

T: And what's that like?

P: Uh . . .

T: What comes up? When you consider that, when you take that in as a new possibility? Are you . . . ?

P: It makes it more manageable.

T: Uh huh.

P: Possibly. I feel like kind of . . . a little free from it . . . freed from it, from having to go down that route . . . and . . . I'm interested to see how I can experience the anger if I don't do that what will you experience, be like . . . I'm curious.

T: What's the anger itself like if you don't dissipate it?

P: It's like pounding in my head?

T: Really?

P: And . . . I just feel a lot of tension . . . tightening of the muscles, you know, my shoulders and my arms.

T: Uh huh. Which again is . . . again that conditioned fear . . . tensing up . . . response.

P: Uh huh.

T: Right?

P: Yeah.

T: And we know what the fear is already. The fear is of harm to other.

P: Uh huh.

T: Hmm? What in your imagination, OK, does that anger, you know, lead you to want to do?

P: I . . . I picture myself hitting her over the head with the phone.

T: Uh huh.

P: Just taking the phone and just hitting her.

T: Uh huh. You have that visual image of being angry?

P: Yeah. I had that before, a few moments ago.

T: It just popped into your mind?

P: Yeah.

T: Uh huh. Uh huh.

P: The phone breaking on her head.

Up to this point in the process I had recognized the patient was in a dissociated state from extreme fear. My interventions were focused on making her explosive discharge of affect defense ego-dystonic and put pressure to feel against her dissociation. A small but significant breakthrough resulted.

T: And what was that like . . . and what did that do for you?

P: Made me sad.

T: Uh huh. And please, expand . . . don't shrink up. Sad because . . .

The first cycle of rage-shame occurred.

P: Sad because I hurt her.

T: Uh huh. So there're two sides to the feeling.

P: Yeah.

T: Sad, but before the sadness there was a feeling before that, wasn't there?

P: Yeah, like, kind of relief.

T: Uh huh. Satisfaction.

P: That I just got it out.

T: Sure. That you allowed yourself to afflict harm on other, right? I mean, anger as an emotion, as a rising emotion, just . . . by its very nature . . . right? . . . is designed to mobilize you to create harm, right?

P: Yeah, it seems . . .

T: That's its biological purpose: to defend territory, or to defend yourself against . . .

P: Uh huh.

T: . . . an invader.

P: Uh huh.

T: Hmm?

P: Yeah.

T: So, that powerful instinctual force within you wants to, you know, inflict physical harm. Yeah, what came into your . . .

P: That's scary . . . that's the scary part.

T: Yeah, you're in touch see? There's no dissociation . . . you're in touch with the fear, right? OK. And, there's another side of you too that's very strong inside of you. Hmm? Which is compassion . . . there's a very strong compassionate side in you who felt very sad for the person who, in the fantasy, you harmed, you injured.

P: Uh huh, yeah. And I . . . I felt, when that happened, I felt like I . . . I did injure her. I don't know . . . she actually hung up on me and I just started to cry . . . it just came out like, just uncontrolled . . .

T: Yeah.

P: And I felt like . . . I was feeling bad for hurting someone.

T: Uh huh, which I call compassion.

P: Yeah.

T: Uh huh. Was there any element inside of guilt?

P: Yeah.

T: How does that feel?

P: Familiar. It feels . . . I don't know it feels sad . . . it's uncomfortable . . . it's something I want to run away from. It makes me feel that I need to harm myself, you know?

We identified the first rage-guilt cycle:

T: Uh huh. Yeah. And, that will be sort of like, you know, obviously self-destructive, but how . . . how do you mean to harm yourself . . . in what way?

P: I'm not sure. You know, somehow punish myself for having caused pain to someone else.

T: In what way? What would be your approach, your style of self-punishment?

P: I think, not doing things that are healthy for myself that I need to do. Just simple things like taking care of myself . . . eating well . . .

T: I would think of not letting yourself, you know, be close to people. Hmm? Who are you going to be close to . . . pushing people who you're going to be close to . . .

P: Uh huh.

T: . . . away.

P: Yeah.

T: Good, there's like something trying to break through.

P: Uh huh.

T: A rising emotion. What do you notice inside . . . when you heard me say that, what was it?

P: I'm tearful when . . . um . . . you know like I want to cry.

We return to the nightmare memory of approaching her parents' bedroom, but being paralyzed to approach them.

P: I was afraid of like . . . I was afraid of my father.

T: Uh huh.

P: Um . . . he . . . he sexually abused me when I was a very little kid and it must have already occurred then, and I was afraid to go there at night in their . . . in their bedroom . . . there's . . . may be something sexual going on and I can't . . . and I can't go there . . . and I'm . . . and I'm left alone.

T: Hmm. I see.

P: And um . . . and then that's it.

T: Well that's a lot.

P: Yeah.

T: Uh huh. How are you feeling? Right this second?

P: Heavy.

T: Uh huh. Talk about it.

P: You know like um . . . I've a big weight on my . . . I feel like . . . weight over me.

T: Oh yeah.

P: I feel like . . . I feel a fear right here. I feel like um . . . it's like . . . something . . . it's like impending doom, like something's going to happen.

T: Uh huh. Again, I want you to just notice something . . . that was . . . that was missing. OK? Just like we did earlier when I noticed . . . showed you fear was missing. OK? Anger was missing this time. Now, I can't prove this to you, OK? But, I would, you know, if I were . . . that the anger bypassed consciousness and moved right into that depressed, heavy place.

The second rage-shame, rage-guilt cycle occurred, but it was invisible, only presenting as a depressed mood. After some more pressure to feel, she makes contact with the unconscious anger which caused her depressed mood.

P: It's like . . . burning pot of boiling, burning stuff . . . boiling up inside of me and . . . you know like you're boiling over and coming into steam and . . . and . . . and just a lot of . . . a lot of heat and . . .

T: And it's big.

P: Yeah.

T: And this way you're describing it, it takes a lot of . . .

P: It's my . . . it's my entire body, I feel it like going down into my legs . . . I feel it everywhere.

T: And would you just imagine that anger, OK, and imagine what that anger wants to do if it were just allowed, you know, just like you did with the operator, if you would allow yourself to imagine what would happen if that, say, you expressed it here. What would you . . .

P: I haven't . . .

T: In the imagination.

P: I . . . imagine just taking like a cord and putting it around his neck and squeezing it . . .

T: Uh huh.

P: And . . . you know, him like not being able to breathe and his whole body squirming, squirming, um . . . until he, you know, passes out from not enough air.

T: And, would there be in your fantasy, a desire for him to think something as he's dying? Would you want him to have some consciousness, would there be a thought or sequence of thoughts you would like him to entertain?

P: I think that . . . "Now she's getting me back," you know, "this is what I'm getting for what I did . . . my payback."

T: Huh. So you'd want him to link in his own consciousness your very slow murder of him with his wrongful act against your person.

P: Uh huh.

T: Hmm huh. And do you feel satisfaction; do you feel relief when you see that?

P: I don't know . . . I feel sad.

T: Hmm. And may I ask why you skip relief. I was trying . . .

The third rage-shame, rage-guilt cycle, demonstrated by the inhibition of relief. Notice the technique of re-ignition (attunement to the shut down).

P: I don't know, I didn't experience it.

T: Uh huh. But, please take your time. These . . . these missing feelings are very important.

P: Ahhh.

T: Is there something wrong with that?

P: What? Feeling relief?

T: Satisfaction. Yeah.

P: Yes, because it's not . . . OK to . . . cause something to . . . it's not OK to hurt someone because they hurt you. It's not . . .

T: That's a very strong voice in your mind?

P: Yeah. I . . .

T: Whew.

P: He doesn't really deserve to be hurt. And then I feel sad.

T: Oh wow. So, you're traumatizing yourself. And that makes me sad, that you would abandon yourself like that.

P: Yeah.

T: And align your emotions with your father . . . with the perpetrator . . . 'cause there's part of you that wants to see him suffer . . . there's part of you that wants him to know why he's suffering . . . and there's part of you that wants, you know, him to die . . . to pay for what he did to you . . .

P: Uh huh.

T: . . . with his life. OK? And those are valid emotions?

P: Uh huh.

T: They're . . . they're equally valid . . . to the side of you that is merciful and compassionate.

P: Uh huh. So, I think I need to . . . not spend more time, but feel that . . . kind of relief, uh . . . for . . . for retaliation or . . .

T: To experience satisfaction.

P: Yeah.

The therapeutic alliance is starting to take control of the process and the patient spontaneously reveals more murderous feeling.

P: How about if I kill him in a different way? Could I do it?

P: . . . something more violent . . . that would be more . . . I would get more satisfaction out of . . . being able to swing, you know, like a crowbar . . . and just bash him in the head and . . . use the end that's pointy and just dig it into his skull and his shoulders . . . and then . . . and, and . . . just keep on doing it and keep on hitting over and over . . . and when he falls down I would just keep hitting him. I would probably just keep doing it . . . it wouldn't . . . it would never stop.

T: Uh huh.

P: I would just fall down from exhaustion.

T: Yes. But you know what the key question is: would you allow yourself to experience relief or satisfaction at that point? When your body gave out and you could inflict no more damage, no more harm . . . and I imagine he would be in some way, you know . . . just kind of almost like . . . like hamburger meat or something.

P: Yeah.

T: Just beaten to a pulp.

P: Yep.

T: Would that be satisfying? Would you allow that?

P: Yes, I would. I want to feel like the anger . . . kind of goes away with his body going away . . . his soul going away . . . his death . . . takes away all of the . . . just kind of like washes it away . . . the blood washes away all of the . . . ugliness.

T: Uh huh. And describe that to me in a little more detail, 'cause those are . . . those are two different things, as I understand the body and the soul.

P: I think that it's kind of, you know, when he dies, like the moment that he dies, then the soul goes away and then all of the painful feelings, you know, that were there for him and for me . . . for me . . . can be lifted up and gone . . . and then . . . I could feel some relief for me . . . that that goes away.

T: Uh huh.

P: And clean . . . and the blood, and clean me . . . of, you know, *all of the shame and guilt* and everything . . . and wash away . . . and it won't be a part of me anymore.

T: Hmm. That's obviously very moving . . . the imagery is so, so strong.

P: Yeah.

T: Uh huh. So there has been some shame that you've carried inside?

P: Oh yeah.

T: Can you tell me that? How so . . . I mean, shame implies that there was something . . .

P: I felt that I was bad . . . that what happened . . . that what he did to me made me bad . . .

T: Hmm.

P: . . . made me a bad person . . . made me unacceptable, made me not worthy of . . . of anyone caring for me or loving me.

T: That is awful.

P: I know . . . and that's why I always have to not let anyone get close to me so they don't see what I really am . . . you know? Damaged.

T: Hmm. And, you've carried this, you know, kind of distorted sense of self with you . . . I think your entire life, hmm?

P: Oh yeah.

T: It's so interesting and informative to see that with his death and with his soul leaving his body and going away . . . the shame that you've carried inside of you . . . is pulling away from you . . . and you know what that implies, don't you?

P: What?

T: That the shame was always his . . . it was never yours.

P: Yeah. That's true.

T: I can understand how you, you know, in an immature mind, made it yours. But it wasn't yours, was it?

P: No. It wasn't.

The session recommences after a ten-minute break and the therapist asks the patient how the break was for her. She demonstrates a re-vitalized self-freed of rage-shame, rage-guilt cycles and identification with the perpetrator.

P: Yeah, it would. I felt um . . . I feel pretty excited, you know, that um . . . real, you know, change can happen for me.

T: Uh huh. Well, I'm happy to hear and to understand that we can get where we need to go and it's not probing and it's not rough, it's just very natural.

P: Yeah, I think I expected it to be a lot more painful. Not that it's not painful to feel these things, but it feels good to feel them at the same time, I mean, it's like, you know, yeah, I should have felt this, this is good. It's not like a negative thing. So . . . um . . .

T: Uh huh.

P: . . . and I think previous experiences . . . it's . . . it's been very painful to be kind of like, half way go there and you don't really get underneath, you had a feeling, and like you said, I was feeling things that were . . . I was feeling that it was myself that was bad and I was just kind of re-living that in therapy . . . um . . . so, that's a relief to not . . . to get over that . . . past that.

Termination Session, April, 2002

Eight months later, in the eighth block therapy session (hours 24–27), the patient reports feeling continued anger at her parents. She says, once again, that she would like to destroy them and get them to realize all the people they have hurt. The therapist asks how her desire to destroy them feels physically. As she describes this, it becomes obvious that this breakthrough is qualitatively different from others.

P: It's . . . it's uncomfortable . . . it feels like . . . scary, but it's also very . . . compelling, like . . . that's drawing me towards that, like . . . like it's almost like it has to happen, like it's inevitable. It's . . . I feel like my hands are sweating, feel scared, um . . . but I feel like I really want to do it. And it feels like . . . that calm, or relief at the same time, like . . . it's just like, get it done . . . that it would be, you know, like movement in the right direction. That it would be . . . a good thing. But I mean like, the right thing. So, like . . . it would be like taking really wide swings at their head like when you see someone get hit really hard in the movie and it makes their head turn around, like I would be hitting them like that, like over and over again, just hitting them . . . and . . . just banging on . . . banging on their chest, hitting them really hard with fists . . . I know over and over . . . and . . . when they would fall down then I would just be kicking them all over very hard, their bodies would be getting kicked from around, getting thrown around by the force of my kicking. They would be like dolls . . . and I . . . and, and . . . their life would be gone. I wouldn't even realize that they had died. I would just be beating up on them so much and . . . they would already be dead. And then . . . I just see them like, heaped over each other . . . and I feel . . . I feel a little sad, but I don't really feel that sad. Feel like . . . victorious. I want to stand on their bodies and claim victory over them. And, I see them like lying in their caskets. I see them like looking peaceful finally, like, just looking, like . . . I feel like I took them out of their misery . . .

T: And how does that feel?

P: Feels like . . .

T: When you see them in the casket.

P: Feels like closure. Feels like the end of the . . . story. It's over. That's it.

T: So, it feels good.

P: And it's like, like them in their casket, it's like, on display for everyone to see right there . . . that they're gone, that their . . . I have this sense that they're at peace finally. I don't think they've known peace at all until they're dead . . . that I really did them a favor by killing them.

T: And how does that feel for you? That's the central area of exploration, is . . .

P: Feels awesome. Feels like calm. You know, just the end of suffering for all of us. And, it feels like I'm happy that I could help them.

T: And in so doing, help yourself too. It's not pure altruism.

P: Yeah . . . no.

T: You're smiling at that. Tell me about the thoughts.

P: Just, you know, that I'm really, you know, just taking care of myself, and just as a side effect, you know, realized them, but, you know, it feels good that I, you know, just considered myself and not considered them, not considered how, you know, it would hurt them or anything, but only how I was able to take care of myself.

T: Oh, absolutely.

P: Yeah. It feels good . . .

T: Yeah.

P: To be able to experience the feelings without having the shadow of them, you know, over me to consider or to . . .

T: At that moment in time, since the first time I've been working with you, you're free of shame and you're free of guilt. Tell me more about how that feels to have achieved that?

P: I feel like, really light . . . and kind of like, I feel like a little, I don't know, anxiety maybe, like fear of the freedom . . . it's a little scary, like, even though it was something bad that I was so used to having that cloak on and now it's like feeling a little bit naked, you know, not to have it. It's a, you know, I feel light and excited and a little nervous, and . . . I feel hopeful that it will, you know, generalize to, you know, to all the parts of my life that are affected. I feel challenged to, you know, carry it over, and like you said, not allow myself to go back to that. I feel like that's . . . obviously it's a big challenge for me 'cause that's what's been happening to me all along. I feel, you know, like being aware of it will help.

T: Sure.

P: Just the, you know, having to have now the understanding of the process.

> And it seems, you know, now it's very clear and very straightforward. It almost seems like it should be easy now that I have that feeling.

In the therapy sessions not reported the patient relived the actual molestations, and reported the experience of fear-terror and then dissociation. When she thawed from the dissociation she felt rage at the violation, alternating with shame. She remembers knowing that what father was doing to her was wrong, and confusion as to why he was doing it. The memories and the feelings became clearer and differentiated with rage at her father for his transgression, culminating in the final murder without the contamination of the guilt system. In the first breakthrough she has the experience of her father's blood washing away, not her guilt over the murder or incest, but her shame! In my opinion this supports my hypothesis about the importance of working with shame as a core affect in intensive short-term dynamic psychotherapy. This was not a defense against experiencing guilt, but a powerful transformation of self from unworthy to worthy. It was her father who carried the shame with him to heaven. Clearly a deep process of forgiveness was taking place along with differentiation of herself from him. His emotional and sexual use of her as a self-object blurred her personal boundaries between her and him. As therapy progressed, more and more anger became conscious toward mother who was oblivious to the three years of molestation. This also culminated in the termination session of murder of mother. Note that the parting with each parent is tender and sad, without rancor or lasting hatred. The patient feels her trauma is resolved. Toward the end of therapy she delivered her second child, a son. Her depressions, temper outbursts and anxiety are gone. She decided not to have a relationship with her parents in the foreseeable future.

I want to express my thanks to this courageous woman for allowing me the privilege of publishing our work. We hope it will be of help to other victims of sexual abuse who pursue intensive short-term dynamic psychotherapy for their healing.

BIBLIOGRAPHY

Bowlby, J. (1988). A secure base: Parent-child attachment and healthy human development. New York: Basic Books.

Broucek, F.J. (1982) Shame and its relationship to early narcissistic development. International Journal of Psycho-analysis, 63, 369–378.

Darwin, E. (1872) The Expression of the Emotions of Man and Animals. Chicago: University of Chicago Press.

Davanloo, H. (1988a). Clinical manifestations of superego pathology. Part II. The resistance of the superego and the liberation of the paralyzed ego. International Journal of Short-Term Psychotherapy, 3, 1–24.

Davanloo, H. (1988b). The technique of unlocking the unconscious. Part II. Partial unlocking of the unconscious. International Journal of Short-Term Psychotherapy, 3 (2), 123–159.

Davanloo, H. (1988b). The technique of unlocking of the unconscious. Part I. International Journal of Short-Term Psychotherapy, 3 (2), 99–121.

Davanloo, H. (1988c). The technique of unlocking of the unconscious. Part II. Partial unlocking of the unconscious. International Journal of Short-Term Psychotherapy, 3 (2), 123–159.

Davanloo, H. (1990). Unlocking the Unconscious. Chichester: Wiley.

Davanloo, H. (1995a). Intensive short-term dynamic psychotherapy: spectrum of psycho-neurotic disorders. International Journal of Short-Term Psychotherapy, 10 (3, 4), 121–155.

Freud, S. (1913) SE: VIII Totem and Taboo. London: Hogarth.

Freud, S. (1926) SE: XX Inhibitions, Symptoms, and Anxiety. London: Hogarth.

Kaufman, G. (1989) The psychology of shame. New York: Springer.

Klein, M. (1932) The psycho-analysis of children. London: Hogarth.

Neborsky, R.J., Snyker, E. (1986)"A Workshop Experience in Short-Term Dynamic Psychotherapy." International Journal of Short-Term Dynamic Psychotherapy, 4, 257–263.

Neborsky, R. (2001) Attachment Bonds and Intimacy: Can the Imprint of Love be Changed? In: Solomon, M.F., Neborsky, R. J., McCullough, L., Alpert, M., Shapiro, F., Malan, D.M., Short-Term Therapy for Long-Term Change. New York: W.W. Norton and Co.

Neborsky, R. (2001) "Peri-natal Trauma, Anxiety and Resistance Against Emotional Closeness." Core Factors for Effective Short-Term Dynamic Psychotherapy. Quaderni di Psichiatria Pratica, VI n. 17/18, 80–96.

Neborsky, R. (2003) Healing trauma: an affect experiencing attachment theory model for comprehensive treatment of trauma. In: Solomon, M, Siegel, D (Ed.) Healing Trauma, New York: W.W. Norton and Co.

Schore, A.N. (1996). The experience-dependent maturation of a regulatory system in the orbital prefrontal cortex and the origin of developmental psychopathology. Development and Psychopathology, 8, 59–87.

Schore, A.N. (1997a). Early organization of the nonlinear right brain and development of a predisposition to psychiatric disorders. Development and Psychopathology, 9, 595–631.

Schore, A.N. (1998a). The experience-dependent maturation of an evaluative system in the cortex. In: K. Pribram (Ed.), Brain and values: Is a biological science of values possible (pp. 337–358). Mahweh, NJ: Erlbaum.

Schore, A.N. (1998b). Early shame experiences and infant brain development. In P. Gilbert & B. Andrews. Shame: interpersonal behavior, psychopathology, and culture (pp. 57–77). New York: Oxford University Press.

Schore, A.N. (1998c). Early trauma and the development of the right brain. Unpublished plenary address, Lifespan Conference. "Understanding and Treating Trauma: Developmental and Neurobiological Approaches." UCLA Campus, Los Angeles, CA, February, 1998.

Stern, D.N. (1985). The interpersonal world of the infant. New York: Basic Books.

Tomkins, S.S. (1962). Affect, imagery, and consciousness: Vol. 2. The negative affects. New York: Springer.

Winncott, D.W. (1960) The theory of the parent infant relationship. International Journal of Psycho-analysis, 41, 585–595. First published in Ad Hoc Bulletin of Short-Term Dynamic Psychotherapy: Practice and Theory 2003, 7, 1.

Recognizing and Working with an Oedipal Focus in ISTDP

Part I

This article discusses an important category of patients who present for ISTDP whose symptoms are activated by love or success conflicts. The author attempts to define these patients along the spectrum of psychoneurosis and describes the differences in metapsychology between an Oedipal superego and a more primitive system defending against closeness and intimacy. The author further discusses the history of short-term dynamic psychotherapy, its metapsychological roots in Klein and Bowlby, and offers ideas as to why the specific treatment of this category of patient has not been as well described as more highly resistant patients. The author further challenges the myth that working with sexual feelings is unimportant in ISTDP. Finally, he theorizes that failed empathetic parental interactions predispose a child to Oedipal conflict.

Introduction

In teaching ISTDP, I have found students have a difficult time integrating classical psycho-analytic ideas about the Oedipal Complex and the development of psychopathology with Davanloo's (1978, 1979, 1980, 1988b, c, 1990) system of intensive short-term dynamic psychotherapy. Some of this confusion emanates because Davanloo (1995a) himself has never clearly delineated the different approaches he used when he determined that the underlying pathology was Oedipally based versus attachment-based. The purpose of this paper is to describe the treatment of an Oedipal case and to discuss differences in the processes between the disturbed attachment cases and those with a clear Oedipal focus. Furthermore, comments and suggestions will be made with regard to management of sexual feelings in the therapeutic setting.

Definition of Oedipal Patients

Oedipal focused patients have usually had primarily secure and loving attachments with both parents. Their adult difficulty revolves around either problems with success in professional pursuits (guilt over competition) or love relationships (guilt over satisfaction of Oedipal longings). An enormous volume of literature has been written on the Oedipal complex. Freud (1913) began psycho-analysis from a trauma perspective, but eventually declared the Oedipal complex to be the central cause of all neurosis. This position has been maintained by some elements of the psychoanalytic establishment to this day. Developmental research has confirmed the existence of the Oedipal phase in children from ages 3–6 and this seems to be a normal phase of psychic development in which gender identity is consolidated and role identifications with the same sex parent consolidate. The Oedipal phase is traditionally divided into two sub-phases first, the negative Oedipal phase, and second the positive Oedipal phase. In the negative phase the female child experiences the mother as the first love object and the father as the hated rival. With normal growth and development transition is smooth into the positive female Oedipal constellation. The male negative Oedipal constellation is more complex as he experiences his passion for his father and resents the mother as a rival for father. However much as the girl, analysts believe these longings and conflicts give way to the positive Oedipal feelings. For the purpose of this paper, I will be only describing the management of positive Oedipal pathology.

Neurologically it does correlate, as Freud (1905) originally suggested, with maturation of the brain and an increased capacity to experience genital pleasure at age three. It is unclear from a prospective research perspective exactly what factors pre-dispose the creation of a positive Oedipal guilt based structure. I will, in this article, propose a measurable set of factors, which may be at play.

The techniques of psychoanalysis are free association and dream analysis and the application of these processes led Freud and other analysts to the aforementioned conclusions.

Davanloo's technique is quite different. His major technique is pressure to feel unconscious emotions in a video recorded interview. From this interview process he developed the concept of neurosis as a self punitive organization driven by an unconscious need to punish the self. Davanloo (1978, 1988) came to believe that disruptions in parental relationships create a deep retaliatory rage-guilt feeling toward the offending parent. This feeling is repressed and converted into a negative introject. Eventually, these negative introjects coalesce and develop a structure or system which we label "the punitive superego" (Neborsky, 2003). Davanloo's (personal communication) major theory of psychopathology grew from direct observation of his patient's videotapes and backwards reconstruction.

Interestingly, his theory corresponds nicely with some aspects of theory espoused by both Melanie Klein (1932, 1933) and her student, John Bowlby. Klein believed in early infant aggression and the pre-Oedipal origins of the super-ego. On the other hand Bowlby (1956, 1977, 1988, Fonagy, 2001) believed in the concept of a developmental trajectory which was encouraged by supportive parental relationships. He also suggested that actual disruption of these supportive relationships and/ or untoward life events could occur at any time, and could cause psychopathology.

Eventually, Klein and Bowlby had a falling out over these divergent theoretical models that resulted in John's expulsion from the British Psychoanalytic Society. (Groskruth, 1987). The dispute revolved around the role of actual life experience on the development of neurosis. Traditional Kleinian thought has several key concepts: she saw mental structures as arising out of a variety of internal objects (fantasies about people in the infant's life), which change in character as the child develops from infancy. The infant's fantasies are only partially modified by actual experiences of interaction with the environment. In her work with children, she was impressed that the children she analyzed had extremely ruthless sadistic fantasies about which they characteristically felt very guilty and anxious. Klein (1935) assumed that the infant's self is, in the beginning, constantly threatened by destruction from within by the aggressive drive—Freud's—death instinct (Freud, 1920). She also saw the child as frightened by destruction from without through projection of his/her own impulses into the mother.

In the Kleinian model, the human psyche has two positions: the paranoid-schizoid (P-S) and the depressive (Klein, 1935/1975). In the P-S position. The relationship to the object (the caregiver) is to a part object, split into a persecutory and idealized relationship, and the ego (the self) is similarly split. In the depressive position, the relationship is to an integrated parental image. The individual recognizes his or her destructive wishes to the object. This brings with it a certain characteristic sadness (hence the term "the depressed position") (Winnicott, 1960), but, correspondingly, the ego is integrated. In the P-S position, the person moves between states of exaggerated perception of goodness (idealization of self and similarly extreme persecutory perception of both self and other as bad). In the early depressive position, primitive envy (Klein, 1957) represents a particularly malignant form of instinctual aggression, which arouses a premature expression of depressive anxiety about damage to the good object. In this regard, Davanloo (1990, p 167) writes: "In the first few months of life it seems that the child expects impulses of an equally primitive and ruthless kind to be directed back at him either from the outside world or from inside himself, which gives rise to what Melanie Klein calls "persecutory anxiety." These impulses thus form a kind of primitive superego. At about the age of six months, however, there is a major change, which accompanies the dawning awareness of the mother as another person. Then persecutory anxiety gives way to "depressive anxiety," fear is replaced by guilt and concern."

So Davanloo (1991, oral communication) shares a Kleinian perspective on the development of the superego. He sees his high resistant patients as suffering from a variant of the depressed position *i.e.,* sad and guilty over the destruction of the object. Ironically, Davanloo (1990, p 190) also shares a remarkable similarity with Bowlby (1977, 1988) when he writes: ". . . Of course Oedipal conflicts are a major source of guilt, and in the clinical material presented here there is no doubt that murderous impulses toward the father in male patients, and toward the mother in female patients, play a prominent part. But where the father has been punitive and the mother passive and distant, as in the case of the German Architect, the murderous impulses would seem to be more obviously explained as retaliation for the father's sadism rather than an expression of rivalry for the mother. Moreover, in cases such as the Woman who Bruised her Thigh, the murderous impulses indeed had their origin in a situation of jealousy and rivalry, but one that had nothing whatever to do with the Oedipus situation, namely the threat of being displaced in the mother's affection by the birth of a sibling; and, since this event actually occurred when the patient was thirteen months old, it long pre-dated what Freud, though not Melanie Klein, would regard as the Oedipal period."

In that paragraph, he has unknowingly healed the split between Klein and Bowlby by integrating the role of *actual* relationship into the pathology of the superego.

It is impossible over-emphasize the differences between Davanloo's approach and that of classical psychoanalysis. Yet he relies heavily on psychoanalytic theory to explain his treatment approach. However, Davanloo in the same page (1990, p 190) also completely rejects Freud's concept of the superego as the heir of the Oedipal complex: "It seems that Freud believed the superego to develop relatively late, and to be invariably bound up in both sexes with the Oedipus complex. In his last major work, An Outline of Psycho-Analysis (Freud, 1940 p 205) he wrote: "The superego is in fact the heir to the Oedipus complex and is only established after that complex has been disposed of." The implication of this statement is that the only source of guilt in human beings consists of incestuous feelings for the parent of the opposite sex and hostile rivalry for the parent of the same sex. Our systematic research data using the technique of the unlocking of the unconscious surely demonstrates that this view is quite erroneous.

Freud's narrow view of the origin of the superego is surely one of those that should be assigned to the historical museum." (Davanloo 1990 p 190)

Here Davanloo again states a position from what I call the "re-united Klein-Bowlby camp" in which he sees a continuum between the pre-Oedipal origin of the superego in combination with "what actually happened is very important in the etiology of neurosis." Other classical schools ignore the relevance of events and emphasize unconscious fantasy as etiologic. Despite his disparagement of Freudian Oedipal Guilt as pathogenic of all neurosis, this *does not mean* that it is not etiologic of some neurosis. These patients seek treatment as well as others with other more primitive superegos. To add irony is the observation that these patients were the original population studied as ideal candidates for short-term dynamic psychotherapy by Balint (1972), Malan (1976), and also Sifneos (1972). In modern practice, they have seemingly been abandoned in the teaching of our art.

The problem remains, how do we treat patients who have a primarily Oedipal focus in ISTDP? Do we ignore their guilt or what? Davanloo gives some advice on this topic in the chapter, "Clinical Manifestations of Superego Pathology II." (Davanloo, 1990). He presents a vignette of the short-term treatment of a man who stopped having sex with his newly wedded wife. He takes the history and notes a wonderful collaboration and low resistance with high motivation. The man reports he substituted masturbation for sex. Davanloo pushes for the fantasy which the patient has during sex and then hits a wall. The patient can only state "I masturbated with my hand." The patient becomes vague, detached, passive and anxious, and he moves into a trial model where the patient attacks him "like a punching bag." Following the explosion of anger the patient discloses masturbation fantasies of "a well shaped, large breasted, dark haired woman with large breasts." The disturbance apparently was resolved when Davanloo linked the fantasy with the patient's mother. He states, "with no return of the resistance the process moves to the interpretation of the patient's nuclear conflict which is an Oedipal triangular one."

This plus a few other selected articles are the entire writing on an Oedipal focus. This leaves the ISTDP student with very few guidelines for recognizing Oedipal patients and very few instructions for the working through of their difficulties. In truth, even though patients who present with primarily Oedipal foci and report supportive attachments frequently have unresolved trauma within one or another axis of their parental relationships. Parents with unresolved trauma are likely to respond to their child's Oedipal strivings with attachment failure and become either counter seductive or counter hostile (Kohut, 1977) Such reactions produce isolated sexual fixation or destructive aggression. From this frame of reference castration anxiety and penis envy are imposed from empathic and attunement failures rather than constitutional predispositions to Oedipal experiences.

So this writing by Kohut encourages me to state that the pieces of Davanloo's case which are not reported are essential. My questions are 1) how was the aggression in the transference resolved between father and son? 2) how was the patient after the linkage able to release the isolated sexual fixation to his dark haired mother, and 3) what was her developmental role in producing it? In the case vignette reported, I believe elements of the superego were activated when Davanloo pressured for the masturbation fantasy as he threatened the patient's sexual possession of his mother. Davanloo became "the father" trying to take away the patient's sexual pleasure with his mother, thus the patient's desire to beat him "like he was a punching bag." Why not explore the beaten and perhaps murdered body of the therapist and see the father's eyes? It would be fun to have this discussion with Davanloo, if he were available, himself so that he could answer these questions. However, I feel that in his competition with Freud, he minimized the destructive effect of an Oedipal superego. Although not as harsh as those of our high resistant patients, these patients can be highly self destructive, enormously self-punitive and self-defeating.

In working with patients with an Oedipal focus I find there are 5 critical therapeutic tasks that need to be accomplished in the treatment in order to free the patients of their problem.

1. They must experience the aggression towards the same sex parent to its full extent. (Pre-Oedipal or primitive superego may be present in more complicated cases as I will demonstrate)
2. They must fully experience and acknowledge the sexual feeling towards the parent of the opposite sex.
3. They must of their own volition return the parent to the spouse.
4. They must experience grief for lost opportunities with and possibly positive feelings towards the same sex parent.
5. They must say a final goodbye to the possessively loved Oedipal figure.

Since most fixated Oedipal sexual strivings are frequently of highly possessive and narcissistic nature, their unlocking will expose even more unresolved needs for attention, admiration, and adoration (mirroring). The pain of these unfulfilled attachment longings need to be felt and worked through in the process of saying goodbye.

Difficulties with the ISTDP Model and Oedipal Patients

One of the most important and illusive skills of ISTDP to master is that of "selecting and maintaining the focus." In thinking about my work as well as watching the tapes of my students, I have developed an interest in how the correct focus is selected. The importance of finding the correct initial focus cannot be over-stated. Since ISTDP is a structured psychotherapy in which the therapist selects the focus to be explored, it is essential to master this skill, if one is to learn the practice of ISTDP with the broadest spectrum of cases possible.

In highly resistant patients with a high degree of super-ego pathology the unlocking mechanism will be in the transference. Davanloo (1988c) has written and I strongly agree that these patients have a resistance against emotional closeness because of the history of attachment failures (disappointments in others) as well as a high degree of unconscious anger. The triggering mechanism for unlocking the unconscious will be the experience of complex feelings towards the therapist. With an Oedipal patient, the therapist might be tempted to move prematurely into pressure and too heavy challenge, creating a misalliance and thus, the Oedipal focus never revealing itself. This would be a pity as these patients act co-operatively, with an eagerness to tell their story, and resistance only occurs as they begin to face their anxiety over their secret incestual life. (See the man with masturbation fantasies above).

I am certain that Davanloo knew this and I can only speculate as to why he did not emphasize this in his teachings or writings where he emphasizes working with complex transference phenomenon in difficult cases. Perhaps, the discovery of the ability to access the pre-Oedipal superego in one interview was so exciting that he lost interest in the Oedipal superego. He is reported to have done a study looking at the experience of sexual feelings and this didn't make any difference, what was important was looking at anger. Until I see this study published and see what sample on the spectrum of psychoneurosis he is referring to, I categorically disagree with this assertion.

So the flow of an ISTDP interview with an Oedipal focused patient usually goes somewhat like this:

1. Co-operative exploration areas of disturbance usually symptoms of inhibition
2. Chronological inquiry of onset of areas of disturbance

3. Emergence of anxiety in describing situation of success or romantic love
4. Loss of coherence in the narrative (emergence of defenses)
5. Trial model with clarification of triangle of conflict
6. Mainly clarification of tactical defenses (Experience of "shame, embarrassment as cover defenses") over repression
7. Possible mobilization of anger in transference if therapist represents the parent of the same sex—may or may not go to murderous rage here
8. Disclosure of either-or
   a) guilt-laden aggressive feelings towards same sex parent
   b) sexual feelings or fantasies towards opposite sex parent with guilt
9. Understanding of origin of symptoms through C-P linkage
10. Lifting of guilt and increased motivation for treatment

I will now present a moderately resistant woman who presents an interesting mixture of Oedipal and pre Oedipal features in her treatment, but she demonstrates many of the points raised in my discussion.

The Virgin Who Treated Herself Like A Whore

First Session (Ninety-Minute Initial Interview)

The patient is a thirty-five-year-old married woman, raised in Spain, now residing in Southern California. Her initial complaints are depression, "problems of sexuality," and her avoidance of "pain and conflict." Soon after she met her future husband, five years ago, she went through a one-year period of ego-dystonic impulsive sexual behavior, consisting of four one-night stands.

At the start of the session she is eager to tell her story, very specific and highly co-operative. She brings up two issues from her childhood: first, her rivalry with her sister Christina for her father's affection; and second, she states that at the age of three she suffered a severe burn, which, she speculates, is the source of her avoidance of pain.

Transcript and Comments

The transcript begins twelve minutes into the interview, when the therapist notices (while discussing the triangle between Christina and her father) the patient becoming activated with symptoms of unconscious anxiety. This is the first application of pressure.

T: But again, we can make all these theories and who knows when you get down to that, but what I do observe is so much emotion as you talk about the triangle between you and your father and Christina. Is it Christine or Christina?

P: Christina.

T: Christina. So there's a lot of feeling there that comes up to the surface.

P: And it's things that I've . . . there is feeling, because I think I've always tried to put it back.

T: To put it back. It's not working.

P: No. And . . .

T: So, tell me more about the feelings when you think of your father, that relationship.

P: I don't remember that much.

T: I wasn't asking about your memory. I was asking about your feeling.

P: My feeling?

The therapist has maintained a high degree of pressure on the tactical resistance, sadness then emerges

T: Yeah, I mean what I've observed in you is very sad. It's a lot of sad feeling . . . coming up.

P: I'm feeling . . . My father, I don't know if . . . I think I've always . . . I don't know if I forgive him any more for not being there. (Patient weeps.)

T: Hmmm. You're questioning yourself. But won't you have to face the feelings first to know whether you forgive him or not? You'd have to know whether you're angry at him first, don't you?

P: Uh huh.

T: So, tell me as I ask you to look at your feelings towards your father, what do you experience, what do you feel right now here in the therapy session? What are you feeling inside?

P: I've always admired him and I . . . I've always admired him and . . . And I love him. I love my father. That's my feeling.

T: But notice how when you say that, the sadness just gets stronger. It's very strong.

P: I don't know why.

T: There's definitely something you're blocking out isn't there? Vis-a-vis you and him. Some feeling is being blocked between you and him. And then you mention forgive him. That implies you have a lot of negative feeling towards him.

P: Because he was not there.

T: Could we try to make that negative feeling conscious in you in the hope it would give you some relief from your depression and maybe even take away some of the self-hurting tendencies that you have.

Therapist and patient establish the working alliance.

P: And how do I do that?

T: Well, is it something though that you would feel good about, something you would like to do with me?

P: To take the pain . . . yeah. I need your help to try to organize my head and to see where he comes . . .

T: Well, let's start there, with organizing your head. Tell me what you're feeling inside, I asked you this earlier; do you have much in the way of anxiety right now? Right at the moment?

P: Right now?

T: Yeah, are you feeling any anxiety at all?

The patient describes her symptoms of anxiety: tension in her throat, tightness in her chest, and a feeling of weepiness. The therapist observes that these are defenses against her true feelings, and he asks the patient if she understands this.

P: Why . . . you started by saying that still I'm not confronting . . .

T: Your true feelings.

P: My true feelings.

T: Your true feelings toward your father. You're replacing them with anxiety, you're replacing them with depression, and you're replacing them with weepiness.

P: Uh huh.

T: These are things that hurt you.

P: That hurt me, yes.

T: So you're still not putting yourself first in a way. If you were, you would face the feeling towards your father instead of hurting yourself.

P: So how do I face that feeling?

T: Well that's what I would like us to do. Now you have some inkling about the feeling, some intuition about what it is, don't you?

P: Uh huh.

T: What is your intuition? Your feeling you're blocking . . . behind the anxiety and behind the weepiness. The feeling you want to avoid . . . that you don't want to look at here, despite the fact that you're so motivated. That's the irony. You're so motivated, yet these crippling defenses get in the way.

The therapist applied intense pressure in order to lower anxiety and block regressive defenses.

P: They, you . . .

T: They stop you from . . . it makes you frustrated. You see how that happens?

P: Because they block me and I stop thinking and I don't know . . . it's just my head . . .

T: Your mind shuts down.

P: Yeah.

T: It's because of the anxiety. Anxiety causes your thinking to shut down.

The therapist has ruled out cognitive disruption and pressures the defense of repression.

P: Uh huh.

T: I asked you a question and I noticed you didn't answer it . . . about the feeling toward your father, your intuition.

P: I like my father.

T: You have positive feelings.

P: Uh huh.

T: Yeah. But I don't get the sense in talking to you that that is a problem, that you like your father. That's OK.

First challenge of a defense: challenge of reaction formation.

P: Uh huh, but . . .

T: But what?

P: But probably what I think is there, is that I like him and I've always tried to do everything for him to like me as well.

T: To please him.

P: To please him. And, realizing that he likes me because of what I've done to please him, I'm not sure if he really likes me or not for what I am because . . .

T: And what does that bring up for you?

P: As a feeling?

T: Uh huh.

P: Sadness.

T: The only feeling is sadness?

P: And anger as well.

The patient unconsciously makes a fist and directs it towards her stomach. This turns out to have much dynamic meaning.

T: Anger, too. I see. Now tell me about the anger. Let's focus on that feeling.

P: Yes.

T: How's that feel inside?

P: I'm blocking it.

The therapist asks what would happen if, instead of blocking her anger or making punching gestures towards her own stomach, she directed that impulse towards her father Renaldo.

P: But how do I do that?

T: But look what you're doing right now. You're going to anxiety and you're going to weepiness, you see? And you even look away a little bit. You kind of avoid my eyes, you know, the intimacy. There's a part of you that does not want even me to see, to be witness to your anger. You want to hide it even from me. Now think it through, how does that help you . . . to hide your angry feelings towards him from me? So, how does the anger feel? I can see it in your body . . . it's there. I'm not asking you to look at something you don't feel . . . you do feel it. You've just learned to ignore it, to bury it, to hide it, to turn it against yourself. And you tell me you don't want to do that anymore to yourself.

The therapist tries again to turn the patient against her defenses.

P: No.
T: So, how's it feel towards him, if you face it inside? Towards him. Renaldo. How does it feel?
P: How does it feel?
T: Uh huh, in you, yeah.
P: How does it feel in me?
T: Uh huh.
P: I feel stupid.
T: That's how it feels? Or is that the way you handle it?

The therapist pushes the tactical defense aside.

P: It hurts. Because . . .
T: Go on.
P: It hurts.
T: It hurts. What does that mean?
P: Not being . . . being ignored.
T: Yeah.
P: It hurts being ignored.
T: I understand. Now describe how it feels inside. The anger it creates.
P: It takes over you and then you try to control it.
T: But don't worry about that. Tell me what it feels like when it takes over you. That's the key issue. You put your finger right on it. And let's not worry about controlling it in here. Matter of fact, I would encourage you to do quite the opposite—is not to control it. Not worry about that. Because all the anxiety is over loss of control of your anger, isn't it? Your fear of losing control with that anger or energy towards him. But can, again, feel the anger in your father's direction.
P: Feel angry towards him?
T: Yeah. You're smiling a little at the idea of it. Come on, be straight with me. What happens when you consider that option? Was anxiety in the about that? Does it scare you?

P: It scares me a bit.

T: Yeah, I can tell. Now you could freeze in that fear, or you could take action on your own behalf, to have the courage to face your anger towards him with me. It will make a great deal of difference in your life. Or you could remain stuck and frozen.

The unconscious communication deepens . . . and the therapist applies a gentle head-on collision.

P: No, I don't want that.

T: So, something already happened. You already thought of something.

P: Of something?

T: Yeah, where you put the anger in your father's direction. If you don't turn it on you. Don't displace it on anyone else. This is so crucial to you to making you well.

P: And how do I feel angry with him, how do I do it?

T: Why are you making yourself helpless again? I don't understand. I see the punch go to your stomach. It's not helpful. How do you make the anger go towards him? That's the key question. How do we break this pattern . . . of turning your anger towards him against you? So, how's it feel then . . . the feeling of being unwanted, of being unimportant, not being significant.

P: It hurts.

T: So what does it raise inside? If you're truthful, what does it raise inside? Without indulging yourself in this crippling behavior of weepiness, anxiety, of helplessness—all of these things that are designed to sabotage your life.

P: If I was angry?

T: Yeah.

P: I almost feel relief.

The impulse was experienced and we are home free.

T: Uh huh. Tell me about the angry feeling. I agree with you. Tell me about it.

P: It's not fair that he . . . It's not a question of being fair or not, but . . .

T: Don't sit in judgment; just tell me about the feeling of anger towards him. There's no need to judge here. I can see it go through your body—it goes to your hands. Don't you feel it there?

P: Yeah.

T: The energy's there. It goes right here to your hands, doesn't it? What would your hands like to do . . . to express the anger?

P: The anger . . . it's this.

T: Uh huh. And what do the hands want to do with the anger?

P: Probably just hit him. (She makes a weak, slapping gesture.)

T: That's not the anger. That's limp. Yeah, what is that? A fist?

P: Yes.

T: So tell me what the fist, the angry fist wants to do. Not you, now, the angry fist.

P: It wants to punch him.

T: If it's set free to do whatever it wants to do. If you set this part of you free . . . totally free. Tell me what your mind pictures that fist doing—how you see it.

P: That I'm angry with him.

T: I know. But tell me, you said it felt good in a way.

P: I see . . .

T: You see what?

P: I see wanting to punch him. To ask why?

T: Yeah, but, in this moment here with me, indulge yourself and let yourself lose complete control of all the anger, all the hurt, you know, all the rage. How do you see it coming out of you, you know, in a totally out of control way—no inhibitions, no concern for him, only just for the anger. Now all of that energy that's in there, see, that scares you. You're still holding back, you see? Which makes me sad for you. I don't want to see you do this. There's no reason that you have to turn this energy against you. So what are you afraid that that anger would do?

P: I don't know . . .

T: I know, I know you don't. That's the issue, isn't it?

With further pressure to feel, the patient admits that, as she imagines killing her father, she experiences deep sexual arousal. The therapist observes that rather than face her murderous feelings, she channels them into sexual excitement. The patient then imagines choking her father, but has trouble visualizing what that would look like.

T: Stay with experience and tell me about it, how it feels. Don't leave it, OK? Your hands are wringing now. I don't understand why your hands are wringing so. Conflict of some sort? You see how you're taking the power from you away? You see how you're making yourself into a cripple? Before our eyes you went from power to a crippled woman. Do you deserve to be a crippled woman for having murderous feeling towards a father who ignored you? Tell me what's coming up, there's so much emotion in your face . . . I wish you could see it, it's . . .

The patient winces with pain.

T: Tell me about what you're experiencing inside. What are you fighting? You're fighting something by yourself. What are you fighting? A negative feeling towards yourself?

P: Yeah.

T: That's what I saw. And you feel it?

P: I feel it (point to her womb) here as well.

T: In your womb, you've internalized it in your womb? Your negative feeling . . .

P: I don't know why.

T: Yeah. But what do you think that is? I mean, we're talking about the murderous power towards . . .

P: It's here . . . (Points again to her womb)

T: And the negative feeling is there. What do you got in there? Bring it out, come on. Feel it. Come on, like a woman. What's the feeling? Don't put it into your uterus. You don't want this dumped to your body. Do you want this dumped to your body?

P: No, I don't. I want to take it out. It comes here and from . . . and it's almost . . . I don't know why, but again I'm doing what I did before, going from the struggling from . . . to the sexual and hurting here.

The somatic experience of unconscious guilt.

T: So there's a strong surge of sexual feeling. Instead of being positive, you're making it into something negative aren't you? So, you see how much of you is suppressed? Now could you look at your father as a corpse, can you see him?

P: Can I see him what?

T: As a corpse. As a dead body.

Communication from the unconscious therapeutic alliance.

P: I've seen him in dreams.

T: You've seen him in your dreams as a dead body? And how does he appear?

P: He's there . . . I see my mother crying a lot.

T: So if you killed your father you would hurt your mother is what you said. This would be something that would cause her great pain? So you would have to keep these feelings of anger toward your father secret.

Insecure attachment with mother from empathic failure.

P: Yeah.

T: I see you both wringing your hands and smiling at the same time. What is going on?

P: It's coming from the peace of saying it.

T: Yeah, that's what I want to understand. What is your experience of saying it?

P: 'Cause it's realizing . . .

T: Uh huh, realizing what?

P: That's I've never said . . . I remember saying it to my mother.

T: You had to keep your angry feelings to yourself as well as your sexual longings and desires.

P: And only five years ago I realized another thing that I wanted to face which was since I was little I would do, I realized five years ago that I would do, uh, always pressing here, doing strength against my belly, my uterus.

T: Uh huh, your womb. Yeah.

P: My womb, yeah. And only five years ago or something, I realized that that was masturbating . . . I'd been masturbating. My mother always told me that that was wrong, I couldn't do it. I shouldn't to it. I'm always fighting . . . (Patient cries)

T: That's very sad. There's a lot of sadness.

P: I always thought that I was doing something wrong, that I shouldn't do it. But then it was . . . it would come to me and I just felt like doing. So, I've always struggled with wanting to do it but thinking that it was something wrong.

T: But help me understand why you're so sad right now, why are you crying?
P: Why am I crying?
T: Yeah.
P: Because I feel stupid.
T: You feel stupid?
P: I've been feeling bad for not . . .
T: About what?
P: I feel stupid for not trying, not wanting to try to know what was I doing.
T: Uh huh. But it seems to me that what you were trying to do was to please yourself and to satisfy your sexual feelings which were not talked about. And then your mother didn't inquire into or share with you, you know, discussion of sexuality. She told you to shame your sexual or to suppress your sexuality, didn't she? She said what you were doing was wrong.
P: Yeah, she did.
T: Which then, it seems to me, traumatizes you, puts you in a traumatized state where you feel conflicted of your own instincts. You're looking at your own desires as somehow . . .
P: And feeling that they were bad.
T: They were bad.

The session ends with the therapist clarifying for the patient that she had fused her sexual and angry feelings for her father. She thus experienced unconscious guilt over either her murderous or incestual feelings, and the complex was somatized as pain in her uterus.

He further tells her that when she feel in love with her husband, this reactivated her unconscious Oedipal longing and created intolerable pressure inside her which she discharged by ego-dystonic sexual behavior both pleasing herself and degrading herself in the four one-night stands.

Second session

The therapist begins the second session by asking how the patient reacted to their first meeting two weeks ago.

P: On Monday I was feeling really good. I was controlling my anxiety. I had a situation at work and instead of stressing I went outside, had a cigarette and came back, and I was calm and dealt with it, with my husband . . .
T: That's very positive.

P: With my husband for the first time in my life I had an orgasm. I've never had. And so I felt good and I was not thinking of anything but . . . it was just . . . I felt that it was unblocked and suddenly I realized that I had it and it was a very good feeling. And then the last two or three days I've just been nervous and . . . panicking.

T: You have? There's been an increase of feeling?

P: Not the anxiety. I feel like . . . I've had situations through this period that I've noticed or I'm aware that it's coming and I tried to control it. But I was, the last two days, not trying to think about anything but just a little bit tense and trying to organize what's been happening with me and seeing where is it going?

T: Excellent. And then your understanding of the anxiety?

P: And then being . . . another thing I've realized is that I can't do everything at the same time and things do take time.

In part two of this article, I will report the unlocking of the repressed Oedipal feelings in therapy session number five, and make specific suggestions for the working through of Oedipal fixations. I will also review the available literature on the effect of attachment on Oedipal configurations.

BIBLIOGRAPHY

Balint, M., Ornstein, P.H., & Balint, E. (1972). Focal psychotherapy. New York, Ronald Press.

Bowlby, J. (1956). The growth of the independent child. Royal Soc. of Health Journal, 76, 587–591.

Bowlby, J. (1977). The making and breaking of affectional bonds: II Some principles of psychotherapy. British Journal of Psychiatry, 190, 421–431.

Bowlby, J. (1988). A secure base: Parent-child attachment and healthy human development. London, Routledge.

Davanloo, H. (1978). Basic principles and techniques in short-term dynamic psychotherapy. New York, Spectrum.

Davanloo, H. (April 1979), Technique of short-term dynamic psychotherapy. The psychiatric clinics of North America, Vol. 2, No. 1. Philadelphia, PA, W. B. Saunders.

Davanloo, H. (1980). Short-term dynamic psychotherapy. New York, Jason Aronson.

Davanloo, H. (1984). Short-term dynamic psychotherapy. In: Comprehensive Textbook of Psychiatry (4th ed., chap. 29.11), H. Kaplan and B. Sadock (Eds.). Baltimore, MD: William & Willkins.

Davanloo, H. (1988a). Clinical manifestations of superego pathology. Part II. The resistance of the superego and the liberation of the paralyzed ego. International Journal of Short-Term Psychotherapy, 3, 1–24.

Davanloo, H. (1988b). The technique of unlocking the unconscious. Part II Partial unlocking of the unconscious. International Journal of Short-Term Psychotherapy, 3 (2), 123–159.

Davanloo, H. (1988b). The technique of unlocking of the unconscious. Part I International Journal of Short-Term Psychotherapy, 3 (2), 99–121.

Davanloo, H. (1988c). The technique of unlocking of the unconscious. Part II Partial unlocking of the unconscious. International Journal of Short-Term Psychotherapy, 3 (2), 123–159.

Davanloo, H. (1990). Clinical Manifestations of Superego Pathology I and II. Unlocking the Unconscious. Chichester: Wiley.

Davanloo, H. (1995a). Intensive short-term dynamic psychotherapy: spectrum of psycho-neurotic disorders. International Journal of Short-Term Psychotherapy, 10 (3, 4), 121–155.

Fonagy, P. (2001). Attachment Theory and Psychoanalysis. New York. Other Press.

Freud, S. (1893). Standard Edition II Studies in Hysteria. London, Hogarth.

Freud, S. (1900). Standard Edition IV The Interpretation of Dreams. London, Hogarth.

Freud, S. (1905). Standard Edition VII Three Essays on Sexuality. London, Hogarth.

Freud, S. (1920). Standard Edition XVIII Beyond the Pleasure Principle. London, Hogarth.

Freud, S. (1931). Standard Edition XXI Female Sexuality. London, Hogarth.

Freud, S. (1940). Standard Edition XXIII An outline of psycho-analysis. London, Hogarth.

Groskruth, P. (1987). Melanie Klein: her work and her world. Cambridge, MA, Harvard University Press.

Klein, M (1932). The psycho-analysis of children. London, Hogarth.

Klein, M (1933). The early development of the conscience in the child. In: Love, guilt and reparation. London, Hogarth (1985).

Klein, M. (1957). Envy and Gratitude. In: The Writings of Melanie Klein (Vol 3, pp 176–235). London, Hogarth.

Kohut, H (1977). The Restoration of the Self. New York: International Universities Press.

Malan, D.H. (1976). The frontier of brief psychotherapy. New York, Plenum.

Neborsky, R. J. Healing trauma: an affect experiencing attachment theory model for comprehensive treatment of trauma. In: Solomon, M., Siegel, D. Eds (2003) Healing Trauma New York, W.W. Norton & Co.

Sifneos, P.E. (1972). Short-term psychotherapy and emotional crisis. Cambridge, MA, Harvard University Press.

Solomon, M., Neborsky, R.J., et al. (2001). Short-Term Therapy for Long-Term Change. New York, W. W. Norton & Co.

Winnicott, D.W. (1960).The theory of the parent infant relationship. International Journal of Psychoanalysis. 41: 585–595.

First published in *Ad Hoc Bulletin of Short-Term Dynamic Psychotherapy: Practice and Theory,* 2004, 8, 1.

Reprinted with permission of editor and author(s).

Recognizing and Working with an Oedipal Focus in ISTDP

Part II

Part I of this article discussed an important category of patients who present for Intensive Short-Term Dynamic Psychotherapy with an oedipal focus. After describing the differences in metapsychology between patients with an "oedipal superego" and those with a more "primitive superego," a transcript was given of parts of an initial interview with a patient, presenting with oedipal problems.

The author proposed ten specific goals for the therapist to achieve to alleviate inhibition and liberate the self from oedipal guilt. In part II the achievement of these ten goals will be continued The specific purpose of this section is to give suggestions regarding the management of sexual feelings (positive oedipal feelings) during the working through phase of Intensive Short-Term Dynamic Psychotherapy. Finally, the author will discuss his ideas on the relationship between insecure attachments and the development of oedipal pathology.

The Virgin Who Treated Herself Like a Whore: A Review

Part I of this two-part article described the flow of the initial interview with a thirty-five-year-old, married Spanish woman with no children who was raised in a loving, intact household, and was the oldest of five children.

The patient presented with symptoms of depression, anxiety, "problems of sexuality," and her "avoidance of pain and conflict." Her current sexual difficulty was anorgasmia, and the patient evidenced that this was cured after the initial interview.

She also suffered from severe guilt over episodes of sexual acting out during her late adolescence. The technique used was that first described by Davanloo (1988b, 1988c, 1990), in which resistance to experiencing unconscious emotion was pressured, challenged, and overcome with Head-on Collision against her avoidance. Interpretation was used as a method of linking together affects, anxiety and defenses in both the transference, and in past relationships. To summarize, the patient after strangling the therapist/father reported arousal and pain in her uterus. This was initially interpreted as somatized guilt over her anger at her father. It seems there were two foci developmental of trauma with respect to him: 1) the father was a busy surgeon who was rarely home, and 2) he seemed to favor her younger (one-year-old) sister, Christina, making the patient insecure and jealous. During the session, the patient recalled feeling pleasure in her uterus as a child and relieving it with pressure. She recalled her mother admonishing her for this and she associated guilt with masturbation, and repressed her sexual as well as angry feelings. This naturally revealed insecurity in relation to her mother and faulty identification with her as a sexual being. She perceived her mother as warm and loving except when it came to her sexuality, and in that context she was rigid, cold and moralizing. The patient's sexuality came under the grip of a punitive superego and could only be expressed in impulsive, rebellious acting out, and it could not be integrated into the rest of her. The prospect of becoming sexual when she engaged with her future husband mobilized her unconscious anger towards her father and mother and initiated her acting out.

In part I (Neborsky, 2004), ten psychotherapeutic goals were depicted to keep in mind when doing ISTDP with oedipal patients. As the transcribed initial interview (part I) outlined the achievement of goals 1–7, this article will focus on achieving goals 8–10.

1. Co-operative exploration areas of disturbance usually symptoms of inhibition
2. Chronological inquiry of onset of areas of disturbance

3. Emergence of anxiety in describing situation of success or romantic love
4. Loss of coherence in the narrative (emergence of defenses)
5. Trial model with clarification of triangle of conflict
6. Mainly clarification of tactical defenses (Experience of "shame, embarrassment as cover defenses") over repression
7. Possible mobilization of anger in transference if therapist represents the parent of the same sex—may or may not go to murderous rage here
8. Disclosure of either/or
   a) Guilt-laden aggressive feelings towards same sex parent
   b) Sexual feelings or fantasies towards opposite sex parent with guilt
9. Understanding of origin of symptoms through C-P linkage
10. Lifting of guilt and increased motivation for treatment

The patient reported being scalded in an accident at age three on her neck and arm. This injury left disfiguring scars on her right arm and neck. The scars required frequent frightening and painful plastic surgery procedures. Once while in church discussing her problem, she was told by a priest during adolescence "this was probably a good event, so that men would be less sexually attracted to her." The patient stated, "This injury is probably why I avoid pain."

The patient had five intensive sessions prior to the one that is reported in the following transcript. The patient showed a regressive pattern of defense demonstrating symptoms of severe anxiety when approaching her feelings. This tendency was addressed as a superego resistance against the therapeutic process in which the patient preferred to be crippled by anxiety rather than face her true feelings. This intervention helped the patient address her feelings in the transference wherein she experienced the impulse to strangle the psychotherapist. The murdered body of the therapist first transformed in her mind's eye into Christina, her sister; in later sessions the murdered therapist became her father; and finally her mother. Each session dealt with experiencing the guilt over these transferred impulses and then the parting from the corpses through a fantasized burial. As a direct result of these sessions the patient reported that she stopped smoking—an act which she came to see as self destructive acting out against her own health.

After stopping smoking, session five, hour six, the patient addressed memories of the scalding in which she recalled as a toddler looking into a boiling soup pot which got tangled with her trousers. When she moved the pot fell and scalded her neck and arm. The patient relieved the panic and terror in the session and for the first time allowed herself to feel anger at her mother in the session—although she never had any conscious memory of blaming mother or herself for the accident. She just remembered fear and pain prior to the session.

Transcript and Comments: Part II

The following is a transcript of her sixth ISTDP session. This represents the seventh hour of intensive short-term dynamic psychotherapy because sessions one and two were ninety minutes in length with each session thereafter lasting sixty minutes. The transcript will illustrate the approach with a moderately resistant woman, who presents an interesting mixture of oedipal and pre-oedipal features, and will illustrate the flow of the process in achieving goals 8, 9, and 10.

In the session at hand, the patient showed re-emergence of anxiety symptoms in the transference. The therapist and patient quickly form a working alliance against the forces of repression, and the therapist applies the technique of "pressure to feel" in the transference. The patient has a breakthrough of murderous impulse and imagines strangling the therapist and crushing his "Adam's apple." Once her impulse is released in the fantasy, she once again, reports feeling strong sexual arousal. In order to heighten the patient's experience of the feelings, the therapist brings her attention back to somatic awareness of body sensations, thus applying pressure to feel.

We enter this therapy session nine minutes into the interview.

Vignette 1 (9 to 16 minutes)

T: Where does this feeling *actually* reside in *your* body?

P: Where in my body?

T: It's all over your whole body, the force is there. I see it's coming through you. Can you continue to embrace it and allow it to push the anxiety away? Let's allow the sexual feeling to push the anxiety away.

P: And now I want to kiss you.

Goal 8b is accomplished as the patient experiences her feelings in the transference.

T: This would be so important to allow yourself to do it. Could you visualize in your mind the kiss? But it all became part of the same person that you murdered, that you're not compartmentalizing your feelings, your complex feelings that have all been repressed and pushed together towards the same person. So tell me about the kiss that comes to the man who remains with the crushed throat, the one whom you strangled and suffocated. How do you see the kiss? All of that feeling comes out of your lips.

P: To kiss is, it's a strong thing, but (pause) it's . . .

T: Strong.

P: Strong. It's strong, it's long and is, but you're not responding to it.

T: Which must create a great deal of want of feeling in you, my non-response to your kiss . . . It's going to create a conflict. It's a problem.

P: Yes, it goes for the same if I . . .

T: Sure, but this would be so helpful for you now. Obviously I know there is no true joy in kissing the dead for the reason that you said, it relates to good bye and good-byes are enormously sad, and painful. Now, we both know that these feelings, these repressed sexual feelings didn't originate in your relationship with me. They're just being transferred.

P: Transferred?

T: Transferred from some figure from your past. You're transferring these sexual feelings onto me, right? Just like the strangulating feeling, I mean, you know. I haven't done anything to you, anything that warrants you wanting to crush my Adam's apple. So call up to see who you recognize these feelings as being connected to.

P: It's still my father.

T: I see.

Having presented this tape in both La Jolla and Milan, the question inevitably becomes why do I interpret her feelings as transference? This allows the patient to differentiate her positive feelings of love and sexual arousal for the therapist as displacements of her feelings from her father. This solves the difficulty Freud (1915b) alluded to in his papers on the phenomenon of transference love. Transference of this sort can become a major resistance as the patient and therapist "fall in love."

After the patient acknowledges the transferential nature of the feeling, the therapist pressures her for specificity. This then causes an even greater rise in affect. The therapist asks, "Would she prefer to kiss her father as a dead man or as a live man?"

Vignette 2 (16 to 46 minutes)

P: I would like that one better (live) than *that* person. (Referring to therapist's corpse)

T: Now tells me of its effect on you, that's what I'm exploring with you. How does it affect you physically and emotionally? What do you feel?

P: The feeling and how it feels good.

T: Um mm. Um mm. Now tell me about his kiss, not just your kiss, but tell me about his kiss. How does he return the kiss?

(Pause)

P: I've never talked about that or experienced that feeling.

T: I know. But be careful, we're going down the wrong pathway here. See the anxiety coming back. Which would you prefer to have, the feeling that you've never thought about or anxiety?

P: The feeling that I've never thought about.

(Pause)

P: My husband doesn't kiss, feeling the kiss. A kiss would be very good.

T: Tell me more description of the experience if you would be so open to tell me. How it feels to let your whole body . . .

P: It feels very good.

T: Actually there's that feeling again to push the anxiety away completely. So where do you feel the feeling, the good feeling.

P: I feel it's mum . . . and I feel . . . in my hands as well and my arms. It's like; it's a feeling that is relaxing. *And I feel the heat.*

T: Um mm. Mamma. So it's very positive energy.

P: Um mm. Yes.

T: And no desire to be destroyed. This is pivotal, you understand. The word pivotal, it is the central moment of your therapy—whether you can be comfortable with that feeling. Tell me what happens as you feel the heat throughout your entire self, that you feel tense, so you said it was relaxed and the release of tension . . .

P: No, I was, in my mind, I was umm thinking of the things that were stopping me feeling it's . . ., the . . ., the . . .

T: Um mm. Do you want to speak those or . . . ?

P: No, well, I can say, but I was just being scared in my mind and playing tricks.

T: The self-destructive force is expressing itself . . .

P: And thinking the kiss would never come and that, that . . .

T: Um mm, mm.

P: You know, I'm almost doing this cuddling in my body. (light laugh)

T: Um mm, which is sweet, isn't it? That's the way I would hope that you learn to treat yourself. So again, tell me again 'cause I'm seeing anxiety coming back to a small degree in your hands now.

P: It is just that I don't know what to do with them.

T: Well, again, that would be a block, wouldn't it? What would your hands like to do with them in response to the kiss?

P: What would they like to do?

T: What would the hands like to do? The energy's building up. You said it's a warm feeling.

P: Yeah, but that's in the kiss and after the kiss, it's . . .

T: After the kiss, what would you like to do?

P: . . . it's umm . . .

T: How would you like to touch him?

P: Now it's the touching, it's touching . . .

T: How? But you have a block, in picturing the touch, and in the touching there is nothing that is off limits, huh? Could you have drawn these arbitrary lines in your mind? Your mother has participated, right? To suppress your sexuality and draw lines. Umm? So I don't know whether you submit to maternal authority in such an obedient way and yet you get afraid when you have a positive impulse to use those hands to express love. How do you see the touch, where do you see the touch? As specific as you are with the kiss, did you see how helpful it was when you were specific about the kiss? There's a little bit of anxiety in your left hand, not in your right. Tell me what the two hands would like to do to express the love however it wants to go with no censorship and no artificial boundaries drawn by anyone.

P: It's umm they call it, this is cuddling?

T: Cuddling, stroking . . .

P: Stroking, playing with the whole body.

T: A little anxiety came in just now when you said, "the whole body." You got anxious about something, didn't you?

P: Um mm.

T: The face doesn't, doesn't create as much anxiety as touching the body. There's something about the whole body that made you tense again and pull back.

P: Yeah, the body's blocked, the touching of the, the penis. I've never let myself place my hands to a penis.

T: Oh my. That's been like a taboo.

P: It's, inside of me, it's never felt like, I could feel strange for me to do it.

T: Ah yes, of course it does, you see. I think you understand why now, don't you? Umm. Cause you're terrified to defy your mother in this very strict prohibition. Did she implant it? Do you feel that was correct to do that to you? That was the right way to be treated by mother?

P: No.

T: So what would the mother that you would, that you would rush to have, how would she tell you about your desire to touch and stroke the male penis, the male genitals? How would you like to have been treated?

P: That there is no problem, that it's natural and it's . . .

T: So could we together push this anxiety out of you once and for all?

P: Umm.

T: So can, as you imagine before the kiss, when your father was very, very responsive, could we imagine how he would respond to you stroking his penis . . . Can it be examined?

P: Hmm mm.

T: And how does that make you feel, when you see him responding to you in . . . Be careful of anxiety. We want you to push the anxiety out. There is no room for anxiety. There's no room here for anxiety. So tell me about good. What good feelings fill you in every orifice, in every space in your mind?

P: It feels good to hold, a body feels good to feel and see the response, the interaction, the feeling.

T: It's very emotional for me, I mean, to see you healing, you know.

P: Yeah, it's good. I feel good and umm feel good, the heat's a good feeling.

T: In your genitals?

P: Genitals? My whole body.

T: Uh huh. And can you feel the reciprocal excitement, the arousal increasing in you towards him? Your anxiety, a little tight, is there a hint of fear there? It's fear of mother's wrath, isn't it? No?

P: No.

T: What was it?

P: No, I was feeling its intensity.

T: Good, oh good. So you pushed all that away then successfully. All the fears. And then tell me the imagined behavior in response to the feeling . . .

P: (inaudible)

T: You see your father responding to your touching his penis with the erection and you feel good, completely good, and what is it you want to do?

P: Continue and make love to him.

T: I see some embarrassment.

P: No.

T: Yeah, there's some discomfort. Push it away. You're not describing anything, anything, to be embarrassed about. Embarrassment is shame. There is nothing to be ashamed of in these feelings. These feelings are beautiful, they are natural, OK, they're appropriate. Umm. The longed for connection, you know. There's some new growth. (pause)

P: I agree.

The patient unconsciously pulls her hand back.

T: There's a lot happening. What's the hand doing there if it goes in the other direction? Yeah.

P: It's cuddling, it's going home. I'm feeling, I'm feeling my body getting more free.

T: Umm mm. That's long overdue, isn't it?

P: Yeah. Umm mm.

T: And as the fantasy unfolds in your mind, describe the lovemaking that you and he engage in.

P: Describe?

T: It's got to go in his direction, and then, umm, as he does with the same fondness that killed him, out of frustration, hmm? Those hands really want to make love to him, don't they? Not to kill him but to, to give him wonderful sense of pleasure, hmmm?

P: I am, I'm so stupid, I get uh uh . . .

T: You get what?

P: I get—there's always the little girl coming like being and the mother and being almost ashamed of exploring that.

T: Oh yeah, but then you caught it. You caught it and you understood what was happening. It was your mother again invading your mind and not wanting to leave, not wanting to relinquish control over you, not wanting to relinquish control over your sexuality.

P: Um mm.

T: And you used to be so obedient to her. As if you swallowed everything she said hook, line, and sinker as being the word of God or something, who knows.

P: Even when I was against her, that was always on my mind. It was there and threatening.

T: Right. It's like brainwashed. Push it away. Stand up for yourself. Stand up for your sexuality. Don't give her that power anymore. So what was the image? You already saw something between you and your dad, when you were seeing the lovemaking, what was the, what was the way in which you saw yourself and him making love?

P: Hmm.

T: Where was his penis?

P: No, it's already inside of me.

T: Oh? Push the anxiety away. You don't want . . . the anxiety gets in the way of the connection, hmmm? Isn't this a loving connection, I mean it's a desire to be connected in a fully loving and deeply intimate way?

P: Again, trying to picture it, it's blocking, but I can feel it's . . .

T: Feeling is more important than picturing it. Picturing in many ways is a defense against feeling.

P: Because trying to picture it . . .

T: Feeling is a hundred percent more important. I just use pictures as a way of encouraging you to feel. The more you feel, the more complete you are as a woman.

P: It feels good. I'm just trying to maintain that feeling inside of me.

T: Um mm. And what is it you like about that feeling?

P: It the calmest I've been.

T: Um mm. In a beautiful way, you're united with a part of yourself from which you've split off.

P: But I don't know why I'm . . .

T: Scared?

P: I'm feeling just a bit strange.

T: OK.

P: I don't know if I want to cry or if I want to love.

T: It doesn't matter. Do either one. You can do both. It's a moment of great significance as you incorporate the loving part of your father into yourself. This separation has been, you know, far too long. It's gone on too long.

P: Hmm mm.

T: You're smiling at something.

P: I'm smiling because I, I just, I had just pushed away the thought of what took you so long?

T: That's a comforting thought or a critical thought? I don't know if it was a compliment or a putdown?

P: Yeah.

T: And what would be the non-critical thought?

P: I'm finally . . . (small laugh)

T: Finally, yeah, becoming whole.

The following vignette shows the patient at the thirteenth session (hour fourteen of her therapy) when she discusses her gains and initiates discussion of termination. All signs of anxiety are gone and her hand movements are now supple and graceful.

Vignette 3 (Session Thirteen: 0–5 minutes)

P: I feel a lot of difference inside of me. I do feel in my mind and in my daily, during the day, I feel it's . . .

T: Elaborate on the difference. I'd like to share that with you. What would that, what is that like?

P: I feel more strong and I feel more confidence, and I'm getting more and more confidence as well in my work and the things that I do, which is something that I had, that I had started not having that confidence, and I do, I feel that when I'm working on a project, when I'm designing, when I'm talking with a client and they like the things that I do and I understand what they want and I feel more stronger and more confidence.

T: Um mm.

P: I feel my, more confidence when I talk with my family and I feel more confidence with my husband, and I think we, we've really grown up this year and we feel that, we both feel that and it's good. We really work as a team and umm, we love each other very much and that's a good feeling.

Comments on Psychopathology and Technique of Working Through

One part of a psychotherapeutic process is not more important than any other, and I cannot state that this particular session led to this patient's favorable result. However, the patient in her self-analysis stated that facing her sexuality and removing guilt from being sexual was the most important aspect of her treatment. She reported the emergence of a powerful sexuality in her relationship with her husband. Interestingly once she and her husband began to enjoy a deep sexual life her maternally based guilt feelings again became conscious. She was able to overcome guilt about enjoying sex in a way she knew her mother never had allowed herself to. Thus, the process of therapy allowed her and her partner to enrich their marriage.

In summary, the therapy addressed the following sources of negative superego introjects for this patient:

- Facing her sadistic impulses, guilt and grief at father for his seeming unavailability
- Jealous rage at her younger sister as his favorite
- Sadistic impulse, guilt and grief at her father for being a source of excitement without any outlet for her feeling
- Murderous impulse, guilt and grief at her mother for her shaming, rigid position about her sexuality
- Murderous impulse, guilt and grief at her aunt (mother's sister) for loss of interest in her as a teenager

The psychotherapy efficiently addressed these murderous and sadistic impulses underlying her anxiety. However, in so doing an avalanche of repressed libido from childhood was liberated. This libido remained as an on-going source of intra-psychic conflict until the process of visualization or "dreaming while awake" as used by Davanloo (1999) was applied to process the feelings. Viewers of the videotape—mainly male psychotherapists—reported feeling anxiety at the direct imagery of father-daughter sex. This is of course a controversial topic, but I know of no other authentic way to help this woman restore the part of herself she had split into her unconscious. Leaving this material unfelt would create future inhibition from repressed oedipal guilt. Thus, working with sexual material in psychotherapy is an important skill for dynamic psychotherapists to acquire.

Why use visualization? Visualization mimics dreaming. Visualization is largely a right hemisphere process. It requires the patient to access somato-sensory aspects of themselves and to become aware of their action tendencies—instead of registering feelings as behavior equivalents which produces guilt. This process of visualization is a cornerstone of Davanloo's method. The visualization of affect seems to push aside left hemisphere dominance and allows for an unusual form of free association. Files of repressed feelings and memories cascade forward from the unconscious mind. In this case the patient confronted her impulses, guilt and grief in the transference and once, impulse, guilt and grief was visualized, somatosensory sexual feeling became the focus. In Davanloo's technique, there is always a very subtle push towards narrative creation about the affects. Each of us who practice this method usually have a fairly standard protocol for working with aggression from attachment failures which involve facing the murderous feeling, looking at the corpse, and parting from the corpse with some sense of repair of the original trauma. This is actually story telling in its most basic form: broken bond leading to revenge, leading to spiritual repair (Neborsky, 1995). We now know from interpersonal neurobiology that story telling serves the function of balancing our two hemispheres and giving us a sense of integration after emotional arousal.

The technique I used with this patient is exactly the same with a slightly different story line: Girl loses forbidden boy and in so doing loses an important part of herself. Girl overcomes fear of guilt and shame and in so doing transforms into a woman. This story has been told millions of times in different forms.

Potential Counter-Transference Issues

The role of counter-transference in ISTDP is another area, which needs much discussion and study. In working with sexuality the possibilities for counter-transference are legion. It is beyond the scope of this paper to list all the areas of possible conflict. Most commonly I observe activation of unconscious anxiety. This is interesting, as it appears the process can activate unconscious shame and guilt in the therapist over unresolved oedipal issues as well. The therapists with this set of problems commonly avoid this area of inquiry altogether or leave the process of exploring the physical nature of one's feelings and become interpretive. Because of the highly charged nature of these feelings resistance against emotional closeness must be monitored and extinguished before these feelings are available for working through.

It is also important that the therapist does not supply cues to the patient as to what his/her fantasies are and thus subtly direct (suggestion) the patient. I believe the principles are the same as working with repressed rage. The visualization is a semi-intellectualized way of working through unconscious affect and detoxifying its anxiety and guilt producing capability. Davanloo (1990) has emphasized that the royal road to the unconscious lies through experiencing feeling in the transference and this case presentation verifies that contention. His prior writings left the technique of working with sexual feelings for later practitioners to explore and define.

Attachment, Sexuality, and Transformation

In Part I, I emphasized the important nature of certain paragraphs in *Unlocking the Unconscious* which integrated Bowlby's attachment theory with the theories of Melanie Klein regarding the pre-oedipal origins of the superego. Herein I want to share the equally interesting observation that attachment theory has a sparse treatment of the issues of sexuality and pleasure (Eagle, 1995, Fonagy, 2001). Eagle (1997) suggests that the adult consequences of unresolved oedipal conflicts might be conceptualized as insecure adult attachments. This is to say that the inability to integrate sexual feelings and loving feelings tend to manifest as some kind of avoidance or ambivalence. This is to say that failure to resolve oedipal issues forces the insecure infantile attachment styles to the fore.

I find much merit to Eagle's conceptualization. Clearly, the patient described above developed an avoidant attachment style. Her description of her early mother-daughter experience was largely positive. Her mother was seen as warm, responsive, and available in all areas accept sexuality. On the other hand her attachment to her father was insecure from the beginning. She felt rejected and felt as though she had to compete with her sibling for her father's attention. Her working model of attachment was fraught with ambivalence with respect to him. Developmentally, when she approached oedipal age he was seen as a great source of love and excitement, but these feelings were not accompanied by closeness in the relationship with him. Therefore the functions which make affect containable (Bion, 1967): mirroring, reverie, and reflection were unavailable to her from either her father—because of his physical absence, and her mother—because of the mother's fear and guilt over sexuality.

Following Winnicott and Bion, Peter Fonagy (1995, 2002) writes: the infant finds an image of himself, in his mother's mind, as an individual with thoughts and feelings. Winnicott (1967) stressed that it is vital for an infant to see a reflection of his *own* state (albeit processed to make it more containable (Bion 1962)) and not of the mother's own fixed preoccupations or defensive maneuvers, when he looks to her of images of herself.

This maternal deficit as I have suggested elsewhere (Neborsky, 2001) creates an insecure attachment with an unconscious Primitive Aggressive Self Organization or "PASO" dominated by negative superego introjects. The opening of the PASO exposed the uncontained sexual affect, made them available to the therapeutic dyad, and we were thus able to metabolize the father feelings. This is the process which I believe transforms insecure attachment styles into an earned secure attachment style. Thus, the patient reports not only an increased capacity to experience and enjoy her sexuality, but also an increased capacity to handle work conflict with confidence and grace.

BIBLIOGRAPHY

Bion, W.R (1962) Learning from Experience. London: Heinemann.

Bion, W.R. (1962) A theory of thinking. International Journal of Psycho-Analysis 43, 306–310.

Bion, W.R. (1967) Second Thoughts. London: Heinemann.

Davanloo, H. (1988b). The technique of unlocking of the unconscious. Part I. International Journal of Short-Term Psychotherapy, 3 (2), 99–121.

Davanloo, H. (1988c). The technique of unlocking of the unconscious. Part II. Partial unlocking of the unconscious. International Journal of Short-Term Psychotherapy, 3 (2), 123–159.

Davanloo, H. (1990). Clinical Manifestations of Superego Pathology. Unlocking the Unconscious. Chichester: Wiley.

Eagle, M.N. (1995) The developmental perspectives of attachment and psychoanalytic theory. In: Attachment Theory: Social, Developmental and Clinical Perspectives, ed. S. Goldber, R. Muir, and J. Kerr, pp 123–150. New York: Analytic Press.

Eagle, M.N. (1997) Attachment and Psychoanalysis. British Journal of Medical Psychology 70, 217–229.

Freud, S. (1915b/1958) Observations on Transference-Love. (further recommendations on the technique of psychoanalysis III), SE: XII. London: Hogarth.

Fonagy, P. (1995) Playing with Reality: The Development of psychic reality and its malfunction in borderline patients. International Journal of Psycho-Analysis, 76, 39–44.

Fonagy, P. (2001) Attachment Theory and Psychoanalysis. New York: Other Press.

Fonagy, P. (2002) Affect Regulation, Mentalization, and the Development of the Self. New York: Other Press.

Neborsky, R.J. (2004) Recognizing and working with an Oedipal Focus in ISTDP. Part I. Ad Hoc Bulletin of Short-term Dynamic Psychotherapy 8 (1), 29–44.

Neborsky, R.J. (1995) Les Misérables by Victor-Marie Hugo: A Metapsychologic Analysis. International Journal of Short-Term Psychotherapy, 10 (1), 53–61.

Neborsky, R.J. (2001) Changing the Love Imprint. in Solomon, M.,

Neborsky, R.J., et al. Short-Term Therapy for Long-Term Change. New York: W.W. Norton & Co.

Winnicott, D.W. (1967). Mirror-role of mother and family in child development. In: Playing and Reality pp 111–118) London: Tavistock, 1971.

First published in *Ad Hoc Bulletin of Short-Term Dynamic Psychotherapy: Practice and Theory,* 2004, 8, 2. Reprinted with permission of editor and author(s).

Understanding and Overcoming Instant Repression

Part III: The Wailing Prisoner: Self-Punishment to Self-Pardon, Depression, Somatization and Substance Abuse— Overcoming Blocks at Stimulus and Response

This transcript represents a condensed version of hours three-to-six of a block ISTDP therapy with a fifty-nine-year old married attorney. He has no children. The patient terminated an ineffective ten-year-long psychotherapy and sought ISTDP on the recommendation of his marital therapist. The patient recently admitted himself to an alcohol treatment center for treatment of alcoholism and Percocet (narcotic) addiction for back pain. He acknowledges that he is depressed and needs help. He has a highly conflicted relationship with his aging father who controls and bullies him.

The patient arrives following an initial session, the day prior in which the therapist worked with him on separating himself from a highly inattentive superego. In the prior session, he experienced a partial breakthrough of sadness. In the present session, he looks tense as a rigid board and wears a frightened expression.

T: You look like there is some tension in your chest?

P: No.

The patient is not used to paying attention to his bodily symptoms; therefore, at the level of response, he is using the defense mechanism of ignoring.

T: So you have some tension? Do you want to address it with me or ignore it?

P: Well, I left my wife in the hotel and came back and she exploded at me because I left her in the hotel. So I just . . .

T: That explains the tension in your chest? Or you have feelings about what your wife did?

P: Anger.

T: Oh you have anger?

P: She had anger too.

T: And you have a tendency to change anger into tension?

P: I think so.

T: Yeah, that's what I think too. You have some anxiety, some tension, and then underneath that you have anger.

P: Anger.

T: Yeah, you want to describe the anger?

P: OK. (looking terrified)

T: Let's explore it together and examine it with precision and with honesty. See if we can get rid of this tendency to substitute anxiety and tension for anger. So how do you feel anger inside, towards her?

P: Uh huh. (the patient is looking terrified)

T: In your body how do you feel the anger? Unless you don't want to explore it.

P: No, I just . . . I don't know.

T: What do you mean you don't know? That is the sloppy way you have of approaching your feelings. Remember we talked about that yesterday where you just kind of don't treat your feelings as though they are really important.

P: She yelled at me and I yelled at her. (the patient is blurting this out, while exhaling)

T: That's what happened?

P: Mmmhmm.

T: Yeah. But you started off your interview today by telling me that you had some anger. And then if you could see it as I see it, the minute I inquire with you about how the anger feels, you put up a wall between you and me and your anger. And you have anxiety and tension instead, see? Do you prefer anxiety and tension to anger?

P: I don't think I have ever thought about it. (calmer)

The patient again describes ignoring at the level of response.

T: OK. Well, could you think about it now?

P: Fine.

T: Do you prefer anxiety and tension over anger?

P: It's better to get it out. (blurts)

T: Mmmhmm. OK. So in order to get it out, we'd have to both . . .

P: Anger.

T: . . . explore it. Examine it. Alright? So how does the anger feel? Inside. As opposed to the anxiety and tension, describe it in your body . . . your anger.

P: I don't know how to put that in words.

T: Mmm, so we have a problem? A part of you that just doesn't want to examine, doesn't want to explore, doesn't want to understand is dominating our work right now.

P: Dominating what?

T: Our work. Our efforts to help you. Right? The wall, stands between the feeling itself. Do you see that as an obstacle? Because you have the anger you said. Can you put words to the anger? If you were to speak back to your wife, you said you did it . . .

P: I yelled. (blurts)

T: Yeah? What did you say?

P: Yelled her name.

T: Mmmhmm. Just that was just one word?

P: I yelled, "oh Pam." (loudly)

T: Mmmhmm.

P: At the top of my lungs.

T: At the top of your lungs? So would you say that it was like an expression inside of rage?

P: Mmmhmm.

T: So the anger went pretty deep?

P: I guess.

T: But I am just trying to get you to cue into the idea that there is an obstacle in you to exploring and examining your angry feeling. Do you understand my words? It is very important that you understand my words.

P: Yeah.

T: That you are putting an obstacle between you and the anger, not allowing you to succeed at the task of exploring and examining your angry feeling. Now do you want that wall to continue to dominate or would you like to be able to succeed at relieving yourself of anxiety and relieving yourself of tension? Which would you choose?

P: Probably say I would choose to relieve it.

T: Good. Good, then we are on the same page then.

P: Yeah. (rubbing his neck)

T: We both have the same goal, right? Now you see the tension in your neck right there?

P: Yeah.

T: What is creating the tension in your neck? Where is your feeling towards Pam?

P: . . .

The therapist has drawn the patient's attention to the physical concomitants of his anxiety and feelings, while appealing to the working alliance and inviting the patient to quit his self-negligent position.

T: Now we don't put a wall between you and the feeling because you said you don't want to do that remember? So how do you experience this anger inside?

P: It's like coming out of my hands.

T: Mmmhmm, yeah.

P: It must be the wall.

T: No. I don't think so. I think that's the anger, it's going right to your hands. When you say it's coming out of your hands, describe what your hands feel like.

P: Like an energy coming out of my hands. (the patient moves his arms catatonically)

T: Mmmhmm, yeah, right. So there is an energy that's getting released kind of out of your hands? Now, again, do you understand the meaning of the word impulse?

P: Sure.

T: Good, good. What's impulse mean to you?

P: Reacting without thinking.

T: Mmmhmm, that's exactly right. If your hands were to use that energy to react without thinking, to express the anger, what would your hands want to do . . . to Pam? Because you verbally discharged the anger, you yelled. But, what if your hands were the expressive for you? What would they do?

P: I don't know.

Since the patient still refuses to pay attention to his emotional response, the therapist uses a low-intensity HOC.

T: See, that's where I think you have a problem right there. You don't tune in to your body very well. Now I suspect that this has been a problem for a long, long, long time. Right? That you ignore the physical sensations of your anger. I think it was good that you could feel the energy. OK? But I think it was bad that you couldn't feel the impulse that the energy creates. So stand up for the anger. Metaphorically speaking, stand up for the anger, see?

P: Well, it doesn't have to be metaphor.

T: Mmmhmm. So what does the anger want to do if you aren't crippling it, if you're not . . .

P: Stand up and fight.

T: Mmhmm, yeah. Did you get a picture of that in your mind? And what do you see . . . in your mental picture?

P: Standing up and fighting, physically.

T: Mmhmm, yeah, describe the battle.

P: Like a boxing match.

T: Mmmhmm, and talk about it. This is very good for you.

P: Just hitting back and forth.

T: Mmmhmm, and would you consider this like welterweight blows or heavyweight blows?

P: I have no idea.

T: I mean what . . . give me some idea of force. Some idea of the force you see in that mental picture. Is it a big force?

P: No.

T: So you still cripple it somewhat? Yeah, that's what I think you do. So without crippling the force, if the force is allowed to be expressed in the fight, you know, to the fullest extent possible.

P: I don't know.

T: What do you see happening?

P: I don't know.

T: I understand that you don't know, but that is the wall. Because it was good you saw a boxing match, don't you agree? That was an achievement, that was accomplishment. You saw a picture in your mind of your anger coming out of your fists. But the bad part of it was that you kind of down-regulated it, you kind of crippled the energy a bit. Right? Because what would happen if all the energy came out in that fight, I mean what would be the ultimate outcome of the fight if you didn't hold yourself back?

P: I don't know, I am back to the blow up.

T: Good, the blow up. And what . . .

P: Yelling.

While the patient moves his arms aggressively, he is acting out by yelling.

T: . . . what do you feel in the hands? Because that is where your energy wants to go, I can see it. Do you feel it? I see it. It's . . . there's no secrets here. What do those hands want to do during the blow up? If you aren't going to cripple the energy for any, you know, for any reason. What do those hands want to do if you feel it? You know, what do they want to do? Be careful before you answer, think about it. Because I want to picture your full force, unrestrained.

P: The physical force?

T: The physical force.

P: I don't know.

T: What would happen if you didn't hold back? If you held nothing of you back? If all the rage comes out of you.

P: It just did.

T: Good. And what did it look like? If we take your rage seriously, if you give it the importance your rage deserves.

P: It's more inward now.

T: Yeah, so you turned it inward, the rage, against you. And why do you do that? What do you think? Why do you think?

P: Afraid to let it out.

T: What are you afraid of? If you let it out, what are you afraid will happen if the rage comes out of you in an unencumbered way? Whatever comes into your mind.

P: Well, I think I did when she yelled at me I yelled back, it was . . .

T: No, let me just explain to you how you are changing the venue here. WE were working on you not losing the battle. And I said if you look at this rage, OK, where you aren't crippling it, where you are letting the rage come out of you with all of its force possible. Then you said, I am turning it inward I am not going to do that because I am afraid. You crippled it again, you see, you turned it inward. I am asking if you have all the energy at your command and there was not a single solitary cell of your body that was holding you back. Picture what would happen then, if you didn't cripple your energy. But you directed 100% of that rage at Pam. And then you told me you were afraid to do that. Why? What are you afraid will happen?

P: Well, I think I did. I got it out. (catatonic posturing)

T: I thought you yelled at her. You didn't use your hands did you?

P: No.

T: So let's focus on what happens with the hands. What's that?

P: A fist, but I mean it is still inward. (the patient makes a fist)

T: Still what?

P: Inward.

T: Inward, yeah, see where we are stopped? You keep turning the rage against you. Right? You cripple its force. You can't even imagine directing it outward. That is so off limits to you. Why do you make it so? I know this problem started long before Pam. Right? But, let's work with her to understand, examine, and explore what happens to her if your rage comes out of you in an uncrippled, unencumbered way.

By this time the therapist realizes he is up against instant repression; he decides to draw the patient's attention again to its self-destructive function.

P: I don't know what your. . . where are you going? (catatonic posturing)

T: Yeah, what came into your mind?

P: Huh?

T: What came into your mind? Don't say you don't know where I am going. That is what a weak man does. What came into your mind?

P: I lost it.

T: Yeah, does this provoke anxiety is the question?

P: Yeah.

T: Yeah. Right. There is a certain barrier that you set up artificially against looking at this part of your rage, the destructive part of it. And you seem to find that very upsetting. It makes you anxious . . . to examine the destructive part of your rage. And you turn the destructive part of your rage against you. Now is that healthy or unhealthy?

P: My mind is wandering. (catatonic posturing of arms and hands)

T: That's ok.

P: Sort of letting myself escape.

T: I am so glad you can see that. That is what anxious people do.

P: I know.

T: Right, the frightened rabbit response, the kind of always wants to escape. Doesn't want to explore, doesn't want to examine. The healthy side wants to explore and examine, the frightened rabbit side wants to run away.

P: OK.

T: So what is your choice, to explore and examine, or to run away? What is your choice?

P: Explore.

T: Good. So again, the impulse is in your hands, and if you were just to let it go with no restraint, what would your hands do? What kind of harm would they inflict, in other words? What do you feel like doing with those hands, rather than just aimlessly squeezing the air, you know? If that energy was directed in an unrestrained, uncontrolled way. I can't tell whether the impulse is to rip or to squeeze, it's hard to read. Do you know?

P: Just lash out.

T: And you have a vivid precise mental image of lashing out?

P: (shakes head, no)

The patient still refuses to draw his attention to his emotional response.

T: Yeah, see you censor yourself don't you? It's really ironic as much therapy as you've had and as much desire to get well as you have, you still censor your inner thoughts and your inner feelings. Is there a reason you can think of that you do that?

P: I guess to escape from dealing with it.

T: Yeah, that is what I think too. With this pattern of escape just so engrained. Alcohol is an escape, Vicodin is an escape. Now you use these avoidant defenses to escape. But what are you escaping from?

P: My own feelings.

T: And impulses.

P: Yeah.

T: So then why? You said you would lash out. But when it comes to describing it in a detailed way, specific and accurately, how you would lash out, that is when the censorship of your mind kicks in and you remain ignorant as to how. That's got to unsettle you.

P: Well, I can feel all the tension in my body. (paradoxically the patient relaxes)

The patient has cognitively identified the three poles of the triangle of conflict and he understood the causality between them. The therapist continues with a low-intensity head-on collision with reference to his superego pathology.

T: Yeah, that's what you're left with. So what are you going to do? Are you going to maintain this censorship or are you going to say no? Stand up to the censorship. Say, no, I want to explore, I want to examine, I want to understand.

P: I'm trying.

T: Pardon me?

P: I am trying.

T: Well you are and you aren't. You are censoring too. You are the one who is censoring, right? Take responsibility for that.

We are thirty minutes into the interview and the therapist asks: what do you feel when you imagine yourself hurting someone? The patient replies "Locked up." He then adds that he is imaging strangling his father.

T: How does it feel to be doing it to him?

P: How does . . .

T: —it feel to be strangling him?

P: More hugging now . . . (strangling motions change to waving his hands)

T: Yeah, but that's a defense; stay with this right now. We'll get to the hugging in a moment but let's not let this anger . . . look, see how you are trying to dissipate it in the air? Where does it belong? In the air or on his neck?

P: I guess.

T: That's what you said. But can you see how the forces of your mind don't want to let you explore and examine this impulse? It's like some secret that your mind doesn't want to unlock. But I want you to stand up for the impulse. I want you to admit to yourself that this is an important feeling and it deserves our attention as much as any other feeling in you, it deserves our attention. Right? And obviously this is important to you for many reasons because your anxiety, your sweating, and your tension sits right over this murderous feeling. And it observes your energy. So why don't you let me help you with this feeling instead of concealing it from yourself, or turning it inward against yourself which is even worse? Why not let me help you here?

P: OK, but the word murderous sort of is hard to get over. (the patient's arm motion is now fluid)

T: What is your reaction to it? Do you prefer "strangle"? I will use "strangle" if you prefer it. What is the definition of impulse?

P: Reaction without thinking.

T: Right. Absolutely. So all that has happened to you over your life, is that you have buried your impulse into your subconscious mind and have put it into your physical being and your body where it doesn't belong. You have turned your murderous impulse against your self, your own being, and you have lived a constricted emotional life. And you're here . . .

P: Can we get away from the word murder?

T: Tell me what does it bring up for you?

P: Well, it's . . . seeing everybody in prison.

The patient is a criminal defense attorney who specializes in death penalty cases.

T: Yeah, go ahead. This is very important, let it go. Tell me what it brings up for you. Who are you seeing in prison? Do you know whom I am seeing in prison?

P: Me . . .

T: Yeah.

P: . . . and I understand.
T: Go ahead, is that what you want for yourself?
P: No.
T: No. So let's just explore and examine the murderous impulse toward your Dad . . . Without censoring any aspect of . . .
P: Regrets.
T: Yeah. Feel the entire feeling. Feel the entire feeling.
P: (the patient is sobbing with a tightened chest)
T: Don't let yourself suppress your feeling. Lets feel the whole emotion.
P: (sobbing)
T: Intense sadness.
P: (sobbing from lower diaphragm)
T: Intense grief. There is a pain inside of you too, I think. Don't suppress it, OK? Just tell me about how it feels inside. Let me help you.

There is a passage of unconscious guilt and grief manifested by deep sighing and expansion of his chest with sobbing.

P: (sobbing) Feels good. (sobbing)
T: I couldn't hear you.
P: Feels good.
T: It feels good. Of course it feels good, it's really . . . so feel it. No matter how painful the feeling is, just feel it. Do you have a mental image of your father as a corpse? What was the image that brought the grief?
P: (shakes head, no) . . . The little boy.
T: Yourself you mean?
P: Kinda.
T: Tell me about the little boy coming out. I want to hear about him. Go ahead.
P: (the patient shakes head, "no." He visibly tenses up) I feel all this tension in my body.
T: Where?
P: Now it's in my feet.
T: So there is more feeling coming up, right? That is your tendency, isn't it, to kind of tense up against the feelings. You see what I am saying? That is the suppression, the feeling, right? So we want to look at all the feelings inside that want to come out. Remember how you said it was a relief?

Because you are letting the feelings which you buried surface. No matter how painful the feelings are, it is better to feel them then to bury them in your body. So usually inside of you, I've learned, that underneath the tension lies a lot of rage. Is it good for you to put it in your feet and tense up in your feet? Or is it better for you to face the rage with me? Honestly, precisely, and openly. Which is better? Which is healthier? Putting it in your feet, crippling your feet? Or feeling it in those hands? Which is better, which is healthy? Because you have lived a long time burying your feelings, you know that. Tension, as opposed to being precise and honest, you know, courageous. Because it takes courage right, to admit you wanted to strangle your father? Doesn't that take courage?

P: Trying to feel it.

T: Doesn't that take courage? It's a courageous act, in my opinion.

P: (deeper sobbing)

T: I don't know anything harder than to admit to yourself that you wanted to kill your father. It's a painful thing to admit.

P: (the patient's sobbing is progressing to a continuous whimper)

T: It's the grief again coming, and the pain. So stand up again, for your rage, be courageous on behalf of your rage and tell me what you would do to the whole feeling, the whole feeling. Not just bits and pieces, the whole rage. What would you do to your father? The whole rage.

P: (the patient's whimper is progressing back to sobbing)

T: Because you don't want to paralyze yourself in grief and just kind of whimper, do you? Because my sense of your rage is that it is powerful. Am I correct? You've weakened the rage already? Now, come on, do you want to look at the rage with me or no?

P: (shakes head no)

T: Do you want to look at the truth of your own rage or do you want to keep running from it? Do you want to escape from it like a scared rabbit? Because a minute ago when you were looking at your rage you were telling me you felt better. There was a better feeling that came. And there is obviously some part of you that doesn't want to let yourself benefit from this. It wants to perpetuate your suffering. It wants to make your life more barren, more isolated, and I am categorically against that.

P: Categorically what?

T: Against you doing that to yourself. Against perpetrating suffering on yourself just because you had this raging feeling towards your father—

I don't believe you have to pay any price for it. But that is up to you if you want to continue to suffer instead of examining and exploring with me with precision and with honesty. Which do you want to do? Do you want to perpetuate your suffering or do you want to face the rage? It's your choice.

At fifty-three minutes the patient imagines strangling his father, then feels a surge of grief. He imagines burying his father with his wife and brother comforting him.

P: (the patient is sobbing and wailing in deep pain)

T: And, do you see yourself walking away from the grave?

P: Yeah.

T: Yeah. And they are treating you as though your feelings are important and they are valuable.

P: Uh-huh.

T: That's good. And as you walk away from your father's grave, how do you think you are going to treat yourself going forward? Are you going to continue to isolate yourself, hide your feelings with anxiety, be cut off, suppressing your emotions? Or are you going to let yourself live life to the fullest extent possible as you walk away? Which way will it be for you? The old way or the new way? Are you going to let your father's way stay in the grave with him, and are you going to treat yourself in a new way with respect for your feelings, treat your feelings as though they are valuable? Your angry feelings, your sad feelings, even your anxious feelings, you will treat them all equally well? You will adopt the new way? You are not going to carry his way with you, or if you do, this burial has no meaning. Do you see what I am saying?

P: I didn't hear the whole thing.

T: I am saying as you are walking away from the grave will you treat your feelings in this new way? (patient puts his hand over his heart and gently rubs his chest) With respect as though they are valuable, important, worthy of examination and exploration, or are your going to go back the old way, the way he treated your feelings? If you go back to the old way this burial has no meaning, it has no psychological importance. This is about putting that old way of treating yourself in the grave and leaving it there. Does that make sense? Yeah, I thought it did.

Fifteen-minute Break at Ninety Minutes

A therapeutic alliance is now present and the patient recalls being betrayed by a business partner many years ago. He imagines his retaliatory rage expressed by stabbing him in the back and eviscerating him. A connection is felt with his back pain. At one hundred and fourteen minutes into the session, he speaks about a criminal whom he defended but whose case was lost to the prosecution. Eventually the actual killer was found.

P: I feel relief.

T: And what else?

P: I can picture the guy that was found guilty.

T: Good. Stay with that feeling. Very important moment. Feel it all, don't push it back down, don't. Don't let the anxiety over the feeling cause you to go backwards. Identify for the feeling for me, once you picture the guy found guilty in your mind. As you identify him. Are you identifying him?

P: I think so, yeah.

T: Good, what's the feeling? In your eyes, what's the feeling?

P: Relief. (tears up and suppresses a sob)

T: Over what? What are you relieved from?

P: The responsibility.

T: But you also started to cry, there was a sad feeling too, wasn't there? Why were you sad?

P: I know. I picture the guy (my client) being found guilty (sobs)

T: Why were you sad? Put your feelings into words. Treat it with respect, the feeling deserves words.

P: I'm getting real dizzy.

Somatization (making his head dizzy) as an instant defense against the complex of his unconscious transference feelings and anxiety.

T: Anxiety. Tolerate the anxiety. It's a powerful feeling, breaking through from your subconscious. Don't push it away. That would be defeating yourself. Look back at your business partner Mike, who betrayed you. Look at his body. Is he alive or dead? You crushed his internal organs; you pushed his eyeballs out of his eyes with the pressure of your blows. Is he alive or dead?

P: He is dead.

T: Dead. So who is the murderer? Who has committed capital murder? And felt relief in so doing?

P: I did.

T: Those are your impulses. Even though Mike betrayed you, you couldn't handle the murderous rage that you felt towards him. You felt so guilty about it, you took it out on you, and you began to inflict punishment against yourself with physical symptoms. Tension, spasm, crippling symptoms, punishing the murderer inside of you. That is how you think about yourself on an unconscious level. You don't have compassion. You don't have mercy. You have it for everybody else. You see? It's all . . .

P: Way too vivid.

T: You direct compassion towards everyone else. You, you treat with an iron fist. And you cripple yourself emotionally and you cripple yourself physically in the face of your passionate rage. You have no capacity to be compassionate towards you when someone hurts you. You treat, you know, accused criminals better than you treat you. So when you start looking at Mike's tortured corpse, you feel guilt. The feeling is guilt that comes up.

P: Now I am seeing the guy I didn't get out. (a disguise for himself)

T: Yeah.

P: Seeing his face in prison.

T: Yeah, and tell me about that. That is a real important image again, I am telling you this psychological stuff is (finger snaps) happening like that: . . . happening like that, so . . .

P: I know, I know.

T: Tell me the feeling that's coming up inside you when you look at him in prison.

P: Sadness.

T: How deep is the sadness? All the way down to your core? Does it bring tears to your eyes? And what would you do for him if you could? What would you do for him if you could?

P: Unlock the key.

T: And let him out? And what would you tell him? What would you tell him?

P: Good luck.

T: OK. Now hear me clearly if you have heard anything I've had to say in this experience, OK? Can you do exactly that same thing for you? Exactly.

Can you look yourself in the eye and can you tell yourself you are innocent, that you don't deserve to be locked up?

P: I am just afraid.

T: You got afraid just now? What, I didn't hear you, what did you say?

P: Free.

T: What's free?

P: That he would be free.

T: Who?

P: The guy in prison.

T: What about you? Because you are in prison too, you are just in a different kind of prison. You are in a prison of tension . . .

P: Yeah I know, I mean I can see it all.

T: OK, good. And how does that feel to see it all?

P: Calming.

At one hundred and thirty minutes, the patient has an image of his mother but resists making contact with his feelings toward her.

T: But do you want to face your feelings towards her with me? Is this something you want to do?

P: Sure.

T: You just, you see, your body language?

P: Mmmhmm.

T: You shrugged your shoulders. What does that communicate? If I did this? That doesn't mean sure.

P: Question mark. (begins to scratch his arms)

T: Do you think your feelings towards her are important or unimportant?

P: The problem I am having is that this is all too simplistic.

T: I don't understand what you mean. I totally really don't. I don't, I am not being gamy I just don't know what you mean.

P: Mother and Father. Mother left. Father died. Mother died.

T: But, do you see, again, with, I take no offense to anything you say to me, but I have got to tell you that is highly disrespectful, not to me. It's not disrespectful to me it's disrespectful to you.

P: OK.

T: That is so-o-o self-diminishing. You are trivializing your experience of these formative relationships. Now that is up to you if you want to handle your feelings that way, and say oh, that's too simplistic (mockingly). What can I do about that? Now I can tell you this, there is nothing simplistic in the feelings I have seen you face in yourself up to now. I think it was courageous, and I think it was significant and I think it was important.

P: (the patient cries, wipes tears) I can see myself burying my mother.

T: Stay with it. Identify the feelings. Is grief the feeling that you are having now? Can you describe the picture of yourself burying her. The picture that came to mind. The picture that you saw, you said you could see yourself burying her.

(The patient wails.)

P: Standing on a hill with the wind blowing, and her body being put into the ground. (sobs)

T: It's painful to see, huh? And how did she die, how did she get in the coffin?

P: Brain tumor. (sobs) After she came back.

T: When you say after she came back, what do you mean? Tell me the story there. The story.

P: She left when I was about 11 and came back when I was about twenty-three and died when I was about thirty-three.

T: And, again, tell me about when did the brain tumor occur? That is a ten-year span.

P: Probably a year or two.

T: A year or two?

P: Before she died.

T: And what was your reaction to it?

P: Sad. (sighs)

T: I see.

P: I couldn't connect.

T: You couldn't connect with who?

P: With her.

T: With her.

P: Because of what she did.

T: There was a wall between you . . .

P: Yeah.

T: I see. But, it is so apparent to me how much you loved her, from your grief. Your grief tells me when you see that picture of her. Do you see what I am saying? When you see her in the coffin? In the cemetery, being buried. So when you said, I couldn't connect to her, right, it makes me think, oh wait a minute, what was going on here? What were you hiding from her? What feelings were you not being up front about towards her?

P: The anger. (the patient twitches his hands)

T: The anger. And, have you dealt with the anger, have you faced it head on and given it the respect that it deserves?

P: (the patient shakes his head, No)

T: No. Would you like to do that now? Picture the anger towards her. Work to come out of you. The anger that you kept away from her . . . How would it come out, in terms of an impulse? If you were to express the anger towards her, what way do you see yourself expressing it physically?

He reports a childhood memory in which she stood by passively while his stepfather hit him on the head.

P: Just going like that. Hitting her. (the patient moves both arms in a passive tapping movement)

T: But, she was a bystander wasn't she? And where were you hit?

P: I guess in the head.

T: Yeah. So in a more primitive sense? Where did she deserve to be hit?

P: Fighting with the guy.

T: Where did your mother deserve to be hit by you?

P: In the chest. (the patient begins to shake)

T: In the heart? Can you picture that and let all the feelings go? Now let it go now to your leg and feel it in your arms. All the feeling. What do those arms do if you stop protecting her from your rage? And you face it with precision.

P: Beating on her chest.

T: How hard?

P: Hard.

T: And what is the impact that you want it to have on her heart? Just like you did with Mike. What impact do you want to have on her internal organs and her heart?

P: Stop it from beating.

T: So what is the feeling towards your mom? Towards her body, when she is dead?

P: Say that again.

T: What is the feeling towards your mother's body once she is dead?

P: Sadness.

T: And what is your verbalization, what is it that you express what do you say to the woman you have just, you know, you just murdered? What do you say to your mother?

P: Sorry we never connected.

The patient now demonstrates repression at the level of response as he becomes stiff and robot-like while his eyes gaze off in a distance. The therapist focuses immediately on his grief.

T: Grief. Grief. And where does your mind go with that? I saw some mental activity.

P: I can see myself standing on the hill, burying her.

T: And tell me about it?

P: The wind is sort of blowing and the bright blue sky and her body's going into the ground.

T: And all the feelings that come up as you see that happening. All the feelings that come up. If you are not going to conceal your true feelings from yourself. Because you are burying the woman, the same woman who destroyed your father. You are burying the same woman who didn't stand up for you when you were being abused. Stay with these feelings. There is nothing simplistic about your feelings.

The therapist is using pressure from the full power of the therapeutic alliance in order to overcome instant repression.

P: (massive sobbing and relaxation)

T: What do you say to her? When she is in the ground? What are you saying to her?

P: Sad that we never connected.

T: Would you tell her another thing? Would you tell her that you have been punishing yourself for your anger towards her and you are not going to do that anymore? That you didn't deserve to be abandoned, that it wasn't you who was at fault.

P: Right. (the patient squirms with emotion)

T: Would you tell her that? And you are not going to beat up on yourself anymore over your murderous feelings towards her. You aren't going to cripple yourself, you aren't going to sabotage your intimacy. You are no longer going to hold on to aloneness as a perpetual punishment for her death? Would you tell her that? That you are not going to continue this assault against yourself? Would you?

P: (jagged breathing)

T: Would you tell her that the only thing you did wrong was to love her? Would you? Will you finally give yourself a son to mother relationship? Would you clean the slate with her? Come on, face the feelings, and don't push them down any longer. What came up? I saw it go right to your neck. What was the emotion? Was there pain inside? Or what?

P: Anger at her.

T: And you are giving it the respect and honor that it deserves. The anger. You are not going to turn it on you, right? Give words to it now, tell her of the anger. Give yourself a real relationship with your mother. Tell her, stop protecting her. Give words to the anger. Don't put it on you. Give it to her.

P: How could she have done this to us?

T: That's a start. Tremendous amount of sad feeling.

P: (the patient is sobbing)

T: Whom is your sad feeling directed towards?

P: Me. (sobbing, moaning, wailing, points to his chest)

T: Of course, of course. Let yourself cry, just let yourself cry. Just let yourself cry. (softly) All the sad feeling.

P: (sobbing, wipes eyes with his shirt)

T: All the sad feeling. Just let yourself cry. No tension. Just let your tears push the tension away. What kind of mother did you deserve?

P: Smiling, loving, and caring. (the patient is looking upwards)

T: And one who thought your feelings were at least as important as hers.

P: Loving, caring. (with conviction)

T: And considerate? Right? One who didn't put her feelings ahead of your feeling . . .

P: In front of me.

T: Yeah. That was the trauma in your life.

P: Now I can picture it for a long time. I feel like beating myself against myself.

T: And what kind of headway do you feel we have made against you doing that? Do you feel like we have put a wedge between you and that?

P: A start.

T: Yeah.

The session ends at two hours and forty-five minutes.

The patient had two more ISTDP sessions of one hour and two hours two weeks apart and then left to live in Europe for three months. The patient returns after a three-month hiatus. His total demeanor has changed. He is lively, demonstrative. Although the patient has felt much better, he tells that he again became depressed, suffered from panic attacks and he wants the therapist's help to address this partial relapse. The patient tells the therapist he wants to address his feelings towards his father. We begin at hour ten of therapy.

P: Well, let me . . . my brain is like going so fast that it's like frenetic and stuff is starting to come together and I am starting to see patterns and all this, so there is a bunch of things I want to go over, but . . .

T: First of all, that's wonderful.

P: I know.

T: I am really glad to hear that.

P: Umm, this is kind of going to be stream of consciousness because I didn't plan, and then we can go where I think I need to go, but um . . . I was really, really depressed, like, the last week in Paris. Yeah. And umm, the depression started I think when my godson, who is like four-and-a-half and his mother died about two years ago of cancer—he started talking about death and it just like freaked me out. I mean I am just putting this together so for like five days I was just crying by myself. Pam was really patient, she just let me, you know, you know, do my thing. And, like the last night before we were supposed to go, these friends of ours, they are not that close, but you know, friends, and they came out to dinner and he was, he was sicker than shit with lung cancer. You know, he made the effort to go out with us.

T: I don't mean to interrupt your stream of consciousness, it is fine, but I want to make sure you are noticing your emotions while you are talking to me.

P: OK.

T: Are you noticing them?

P: It's calming me down.

T: And the, so initially you were having some anxiety . . .

P: Anxiety, high anxiety. That is my one problem now is that I have been having panic attacks.

T: OK.

P: Any kind of stress just sets me off. You know, I start perspiring and I have learned to lie down and rest and control it and I just have to work through it I understand that. Umm, so anyway, when we went out to dinner with this couple, he is sick, you know really sick. And, umm, you know he was so sick, I didn't even say, you know I am starting to announce to people that you know I have been depressed or that I am not doing well, but you know I want to be with you and all this kind of stuff, I mean I am getting much more assertive in my private life as opposed to my public life . . . with the people I feel comfortable with. So anyway, you know, he came out and I could see that he was sicker than shit. We went home that night and I said Pam, you know, I am not going to cry anymore, this is crazy. Look at how sick he is and I am feeling sorry for myself because I, you know, can't figure out how to be happy and appreciate everything that I lucked out in having. And you know, other than one tear or something, I haven't cried. It has been about two weeks. It sort of gave me a huge amount of perspective and so we came back like, that was Friday night and we came back Sunday and Monday night we got a phone call that he died Monday.

T: Oh wow.

P: So, umm. Anyway, you know I have to get through this grieving the loss of a father—I am not through that—but since we have been back I have made a little progress in communicating with him, for me. Pam heard me have a conversation in my public capacity like two weeks ago you know where I was very assertive and totally in control and *blah blah blah* . . . and she says, "You know this is the person that I married and where have you been all these years?" And it sort of, you know, like hit me that this is, I have to tell my father what I think and how I feel and I have always been afraid to do that because of the fear that he might abandon me too. *(Referring to what his mother actually did to him)* So, he called me up, I called him up, you know, a few days later and he said, "Well, I never hear from you and I haven't seen you and . . . umm," and I said, "Well, you know, it works two ways, you could call me too." So I called my father—my father has this thing that if I don't come down to see him only then he is not available. So I called him up and I told him I was going to come down today to see him . . . So, I called my father to tell him that I was going to go down and see him today and he called me back and afterward a few days later and said, "I can't see you on Tuesday because I am having a chemo treatment in the morning and I get sick afterwards." And I said, "You know, that is OK, I will just come see you." And, you know when he shuts me out I get sick, and I don't want to get sick to ruin Pam's trip. I mean, I decided that the priorities were, you know, to make Pam happy and for her birthday to be happy and this trip is like paradise for her. So I told him I was going to come over and I didn't tell him I was coming down here for any other reason because he would, you know, shut me out for that, and I am just going to go over there after I leave here and knock on his door and if he won't answer then I will call him on the phone and if he won't answer it then I will just leave him a note and then come back and be with Pam.

T: So, your father has a lot of power to provoke a lot of emotion—that is what you are telling me?

This vignette shows the lasting emotional insight from his prior session and his improved capacity to undo the defenses of instant repression as he identifies his anger and his fear.

One hour and fifty minutes of additional therapy ensued in which the patient accessed his complete rage against his father along with grief and guilt for his complex feelings. His panic attacks completely abated. On a three-year follow up, the therapist learned that the patient has remained sober and handled his father's actual death, dealt with an estate conflict with a sibling, and a life-threatening illness to his wife without becoming symptomatic.

First published in *Ad Hoc Bulletin of Short-Term Dynamic Psychotherapy: Practice and Theory* 2005, 9, 2.

Brain, Mind and Dyadic Change Processes

The basic principle of ISTDP as outlined in this book is that unresolved (repressed or dissociated) attachment trauma is at the core of psychoneurosis and personality disorders. People who carry with them unresolved attachment trauma are normally high functioning people, but they either become stuck in their interpersonal relationships or develop neurotic symptoms. As we have demonstrated in earlier chapters understanding theoretical aspects of psychodynamic therapy, developmental neuroscience, and attachment theory provides a useful framework to conceptualize the accelerated change process noted in this therapy. Not only do patients change psychologically, but they actually change in their physical appearance as they integrate warded off affects into their personality. In order to explain the combination of both a rapid and long lasting change noted in our patients, the author has created a bi-hemispheric model of psychotherapeutic change.

ISTDP solves the paradox inherent in treating unconscious, implicit trauma, which is thought to be recorded in the non verbal right hemisphere. This locus is largely non-verbal and thus interpretation is literally "talking to the wall"! This is because interpretation is largely a left hemispheric process and serves an integrative function as opposed to a transformative function. To illustrate this point, this chapter contains an annotated transcript of a patient with mixed phobic anxiety and obsessive compulsive symptoms. He is an "n" of one study and serves as his own control since he had a twenty year analysis which gave him insight into some dynamics but no therapeutic change. By his self report he, greatly benefited from a nine and one half hour ISTDP based psychotherapy which helped him free himself from his pathologic attachment to his mother.

In order to describe the evidence behind this bi-hemispheric model there are three lines of important research that are highlighted in this chapter : 1) outcome in psychodynamic psychotherapy, 2) developmental neuroscience, and 3) adult attachment.

Psychodynamic Outcome Research

First, there are recent publications of meta-analyses of many well-designed dynamic studies. (Leichsenring, 2004, Cochrane 2007). These studies demonstrate that dynamic psychotherapy is more effective for a broad band of conditions than waiting list. This means talk therapy based on inquiry, clarification, defense analysis, confrontation, interpretation, and support helps people secure relief from symptoms and, on occasion, change character.

There is no evidence yet that one form of psychodynamic psychotherapy is particularly more effective than any other. However, this entire book is dedicated to describing one highly effective form of dynamic psychotherapy, ISTDP which the authors believe has unique untapped therapeutic potential. This can best be described as an experiential form of psychotherapy that emphasizes the importance of experiencing feelings from one's past in the present as the singularly curative factor. The founders of this approach are David Malan and Habib Davanloo. During Davanloo's career he treated and video recorded 632 patients whom he personally treated (Malan, 2001). Despite the systematic approach the data from these cases were never published. Recently, another author in this volume, Patricia Coughlin along with Malan (2007), used a single case design to study seven patients. Their goal was to isolate curative factors. Their work supported Davanloo's earlier contention that the experience of repressed emotion, anger and particularly grief at a caregiver, in a therapeutic dyad created both symptomatic relief and character change.

Developmental Neuroscience Research

As described by Schore and others (1996, 2001), the decade of the brain has yielded fascinating data about the brain and its emotional organization. This is an enormous area and I will only scratch the surface of findings relevant to psychotherapy, particularly, the elucidation of the right hemisphere and its role in development. Some of us now think of infants from birth to about 16 months as right brain creatures with little crystallization of the left-brain until 16 to 18 months. We also know that small children need consistent attachment figures and become specifically attached to their primary attachment figure at 6 months. We know that this attachment must occur, and if it doesn't severe developmental—neurobiologic pathology in relationships and affect control will ensue. Once attached, the child uses or requires his/her mother to regulate affect. This means that the child, lacking a mature left hemisphere, requires the attention of the mother in the right quantity and quality in order to eventually develop a healthy sense of its self in relation to others. Moreover, specific styles of attachment have been described by (Ainsworth, 1978) and can be reliably measured in Strange Situation study. There are two general categories of attachment: Secure and Insecure. The secure variety tends to be associated with better relationships later in life (school, young adults, marriage) and the insecures drift towards problematic relationships with higher incidences of bully behavior and victimization behaviors than do secures (Sroufe, 1990). The insecure subjects are sub-divided into avoidant, ambivalent, and a more recently described category, disorganized. These categories once established tend to remain somewhat stable during development. The disorganized category has the highest incidence of later psychopathology. There is an increasing mound of evidence suggesting that brain structure is being laid down in either healthy or unhealthy ways.

The secure infant is receiving flexible and highly reliable attention from its mother. These mothers tend to rapidly comfort their distressed children and intuitively give the child "good enough" experience. The child's arousal/stress response system is rapidly addressed and regulated and the child returns to its major endeavor: exploring the environment and learning cause and effect in order to acquire the skills to master their environment.

Contrast this to the insecure infant who is not receiving flexible and reliable attention. The avoidant baby internalizes the mother's desire to avoid distressing emotions and develops a false self of calm, focused interest in the outside world. The infant prematurely settles, but GSR's and serum cortisols reflect an on-going unattended stress response. The ambivalent baby internalizes the mother's worried preoccupation with herself and her infant and hyper focuses on mother's distress, pulling away and resisting affection and thus creates angry conflict rather than relief. This baby's GSR and cortisol are also elevated similar to avoidant infants.

The disorganized infant represents the next level of attachment failure. Bowlby, while at Stanford, wrote his wife Ursala in excitement that he discovered the difference between mammalian attachment and other offspring. "Mammals run to their caregiver when frightened—all other animals escape from the frightening situation." Mary Main along with her husband Erik Hesse have described a subgroup of infants who were wrongly described as either avoidant or ambivalent (1990). They used slow motion videotape to discover the appearance of fright behaviors in the child associated with caregiver presence. Later, they discovered the source of this fear was unconscious threat behaviors from the mother's of these children. Since these children are biologically programmed to approach the parent for comfort/safety they see this as a classic approach—avoidance bind. They coined the wonderful phrase: fear without solution.

The insecure category of infant fails to receive consistent experiences of comfort and care when distressed. Other early infant researchers have described other patterns of attunement failure in these parents as well related to eye contact, vocal recognition and synchronization (Beebe 1994, 2002, Lyons-Ruth, 2002). What it comes to again and again is that mothers of secure infants have flexible patterns of attention and behaviors responses that suit their infants needs for stimulation (up regulation) or comfort (down regulation), and seem to intuitively know when and how to deliver each in the right quantity and right quality in most situations. When this is done correctly children develop solid secure bases and go through the appropriate developmental phases to become both secure and autonomous. I emphasize the research showing that these kids are able to largely navigate the treacherous reefs of school life and friendships in smooth ways. Insecures begin to display difficulties with relationships and affect control. Exploration and autonomy suffer.

Schore (1996) offers data to support an intriguing hypothesis. He states the right hemisphere is not only the locus of unconscious processes but also in particular, the right orbital frontal gyrus is central integrating circuit for aggression in human relationships. He believes it is uniquely situated above the limbic area and this circuitry mediates the capacity for empathy for others as well as modulation of retaliatory aggression. In other words, the ability to perceive the other person as having feelings, and to read and respond accordingly is mediated in the area of the brain. He further argues the quality of attachment, *i.e.,* number of flexibly and successful comfort events stimulates growth in this area. In the extreme, without these experiences, he argues that the child becomes vulnerable to disorders of uncontrolled aggression: thus the creation of borderline, narcissistic and sociopathic conditions.

Adult Attachment Research

The AAI is a conversation with an interviewer who asks you to describe your parents with five adjectives and then to give a paragraph to support the adjectives (Main, 1998). The interview repeats itself with important other in the subject's life (grandparents, neighbors) and also covers losses or traumas. It takes about an hour to complete. The secures are called secure autonomous and their transcripts are like reading lovely essays with poetic language and rich examples. The avoidant adults are called Dismissive. They idealize their parent and do everything they can do to keep emotions low and at bay—their narratives are skimpy and lean. The ambivalent subjects are called Preoccupied and they over speak and are verbally derogatory and cannot inhibit their outbursts. The disorganized are called Disoriented/Unresolved (for Abuse or Loss). These manifest lapses in time sense as well as consciousness. Finally there is the intriguing group of people called the "cannot classify" who show mixed traits but no dominant style. These are usually associated with fairly significant clinical disturbances.

In short, we have a tremendous amount of prospective data that demonstrates that attachment experiences from six to sixteen months of life define what our linguistic capacity for coherent narratives will become as adults. Furthermore we know that these capacities reflect how we think and behave in relationships. Mothers with these linguistic impairments create children with the same linguistic impairments!

On the optimistic and therapeutic side, we know that secures have a more powerful effect on insecures than vice versa. An insecure married to a secure can acquire these linguistic capacities. These are called "earned" secures (Pearson, 1994). From this it is not too great a leap to believe that psychotherapy can alter attachment patterns in a positive way from insecure states of mind to earned secure states of mind.

If we tie some threads together, we can see what the AAI actually measures. As the subject is asked to create a narrative of their life, their right hemisphere repository of emotional memory is activated. The subject is relating to the interviewer while at same time adhere to linguistic coherence. The more troublesome the attachment memories the more pressure is placed on the mind's ability to sustain narrative coherence. Thus avoidant subjects decrease the amount of emotional memory available by narrowing their attentional focus and create dry, brittle, idealizing narratives. Preoccupied subjects loose attentional focus and get flooded with highly charged negative memories and become derogatory, over involved and overly inclusive. with their stories The disorganized subjects show momentary lapses of consciousness that compromise their attention as they deal with issues surrounding loss or abuse because the recall of these events mobilize their unprocessed affective memories. Their narratives are thus fraught with temporal contradictions and linguistic violations.

Schore is eloquent in his neuroscientific thesis that the AAI is an instrument that can measure the health/integrity of the right orbital frontal gyrus in containing the affective data required to script a coherent autobiographical narrative. My research interest has revolved around examining recorded clinical interviews from a linguistic perspective to assess whether an attachment savvy clinician can accurately assess attachment status from a dynamic interview.

Finally, Main and Hesse's (1990) research into the origin of disorganized attachment style reveals a strong link to unresolved trauma in the minds of the mother. Close analysis of videos reveal showing of maternal eyeteeth, sub-audible hissing and anomalous fear provoking behavior. So as these moms who are unresolved for trauma approach their children to comfort them, they are showing threat behavior. The way I interpret this finding is the mom is reading the attachment longings of her child in her right hemisphere. This infant activates the unconscious memory of their parents threat behavior and they are responding to the child as if the child were their own threatening parent.

Integration with Freudian Models

Eagle was the first to suggest that there was an interplay between the attachment system and latter development of Oedipal structures. In the authors experience this is absolutely the case. Freud touched on this in the report of the case of little Hans wherein he discovers Han's mother overstimulated him by reversing roles and thus created or aggravated his rivalry with her husband (see case below). So the attachment system is the basic building block for the experience of latter relationships and determines in large part how they will unfold.

Synthesis: A Bi-Hemispheric model

How do these threads come together in a useful way to understand brief psychodynamic psychotherapy? The outcome studies of dynamic psychotherapy indicate to me that *the experience of feeling that frightened one in the past in an atmosphere of care, compassion and safety* is the singularly most crucial healing factor in dynamic psychotherapy. In earlier chapters we have described this as the therapist taking the position of the patient's "potentially constructive superego." Further the author proposes that the amount of time a therapeutic dyad spends bringing right hemisphere feelings to consciousness the more likely it is that symptoms will reduce in the patient and the more likely character change will ensue. This task sounds simple but it is in reality enormously difficult. Freud first described this difficulty when he noted that even the most highly motivated of us (secure?) resist therapy aimed at recollection trauma from the past. It seems our brains develop an elaborate defensive structure to protect us from a) fear without solution, or b) upsetting our mothers beyond their emotional capacities. I contend that for dynamic therapy to be successful it must overcome these transferential patterns (and countertransferential reactions) to the sending and receiving of feeling information.

What makes successful therapy so difficult to achieve is that the target organ, the right hemisphere has no language. It stimulated by and communicates through images, sensations, facial expressions and creates bodily sensations which we interpret as feelings; happy, sad, angry, pain, etc. Traditional psychotherapy has been largely verbal and interpretive and thus limited in its ability to create rapid change. With Malan and Davanloo's input a large number of therapists are now placing themselves in the experiential camp. Studies of improvement show ability to access sad feelings reduce symptoms while ability to access anger correlates with character change.

Table 1 illustrates the challenge inherent in psychotherapy by contrasting the different way information is processed in the two hemispheres.

Table 1. What Makes Psychotherapy A Challenge

Left brain explicit information processing

- Locus of conscious processes
- Logical, linear (time based), language-based, storage bin for conscious memory, "makes sense of"
- In charge of memory storage and retrieval
- Easy to communicate with verbally
- Shaped by culture and education

Right brain implicit information processing

- Locus of major unconscious processes
- Impressionistic, responds to images, facial patterns, linked to autonomic sensations (feelings)
- Storage bin for unconscious memory and traumatic experience
- Difficult to communicate with verbally (no language)
- Shaped by attachment experiences

Infant research suggests that the right hemisphere is shaped between six and sixteen months of life and is shaped along the lines of Ainsworth and Main's four styles. Defenses surround the profound experience of loss of "good enough mothering states." For these loss experiences to be processed successfully the infant needs the actual presence of the mother's interactive right brain in a state of "care, attunement, compassion, and comfort" Attachment failures lead to unprocessed feelings of unregulated grief which, without the empathic other, create unbearable states of aloneness that can only be regulated with defenses. If the trauma is prolonged, the infant creates an internalized representation of the attachment failure in the form of a punitive superego which ends the state of unbearable aloneness, but it comes at a price. In summary, our patients value their superegos because their superegos are defences against loneliness. They stubbornly refuse to separate from their superegos because they are flooded with separation anxiety and inability to regulate their affective states. Anxiety is seen as the archaic recording of affects that the patients feared exposing to their caregivers. Our clinical work shows extensive samples of patients who have had hundreds of hours of dynamic psychotherapy and psychoanalysis and yet their superegos have not budged. The case summarized below is one in which his analysis failed to expose or deconstruct his highly ego-syntonic punitive superego. Only after the superego is relinquished by the patient, the therapist can become a potentially new transformative attachment figure and rapidly improve attachment status. Preliminary data from an AAI study of patients in my practice seems to confirm this assertion. (Neborsky, 2004b)

The psychotherapy, which I have refined, has a number of sources—all aimed at bring unconscious trauma into consciousness. (Neborsky, 2001, 2003, 2004) Table 2 outlines the factors utilized in our approach.

Table 2. Attachment-Based/ISTDP

- Adapted from STDP and ISTDP—Malan and Davanloo
    - Pressure, Challenge, Head-On Collision
    - Clarification, Identification, Confrontation
    - Attention to Pathways of Unconscious Anxiety Discharge
    - Emphasizes Visualization for processing
    - Dreaming While Awake
    - Psychoanalytic View of Mental Apparatus
- Applies AAI—Mary Main and Ruth Goldwin's Research
    - Linguistic Coherence is Closely Monitored
- Elements of Gestalt—Perls
    - Empty Chair
    - Inner Child
    - Talking to the Dead
- Modeling—Unique addition
    - Therapist speaks on behalf of patient to the frightening parent

ISTDP in part originated from a basic dissatisfaction with interpretation. To solve this, Davanloo applied therapeutic pressure to the patient to feel their unconscious emotions and simultaneously addressed the patient's gymnastics (resistance) to feeling their traumatically based emotions. His goal in each session became helping the patient address the developmental origins of their difficulties and to help patients feel the trauma exactly the way they felt it at the time it originated. He heavily used confrontation and coached, goaded or challenged patients to defeat their own resistance. He believed in taping into the patient's own desire to heal and mobilize their "will" to defeat their resistance. He proved this approach to be effective in relieving symptoms and character but unfortunately never published his results for peer review. However, his students have carried his work across the world and its now in its third generation. Proof of effectiveness is now indisputable. (Leichsensring, 2004) (Abbass, Cochrane) (Malan, 2007) Relying on his pioneering work the author has applied the scientific developmental research on attachment and states of mind to the clinical situation. I also try to de-emphasize interpretation and have re-emphasized the Gesalt elements of the process by having the patients speak directly to their punitive introjects and encourage while monitoring the use of coherent discourse. If the patients flounder, I will model as in psychodrama for them until they are able to maintain narrative coherence with their imaginary traumatizing parent. Finally I have them talk to their traumatized images of self as child in a way that their parent could never speak. In so doing they are creating the inter-subjective experience a securely attached child would have had with their security promoting parent.

This pattern of treatment moves from focus to focus until a critical mass of trauma memory networks are exposed and processed by the extensive use of transference. Once this is achieved, symptoms resolve and character change occurs. Patient undergoing this therapy report decreased avoidance behavior, improved mood, decrease somatization (medication seeking), improved interpersonal relationships with enhanced intimacy, improved empathy and mutuality, and shifts from insecure to secure states of mind as measured by the AAI.

Freud (1900) approached the unconscious from the Newtonian paradigm of his time. We have left Victorian thinking about the universe and have advanced to a theory of complex systems. As we are children of the information age, and the author wants to propose a model of the unconscious based on research, clinical observation, and my own fantasy about how our minds actually operate. We can now diagnose the structure of the right hemisphere with tools evolved from the AAI. Psychotherapy can be seen as the process of freeing the right hemisphere from encapsulating defenses, which, like scar tissue, prevent healing. The right hemisphere difficulties are diagnosed by observing the defenses mobilized as the patient attempts to explore their unconscious affects as well as the general physiologic patterns of the patient's anxiety. Is the majority of the anxiety held in striated muscle pathways as tension (secure pattern) or is the anxiety pathway primarily parasympathetically mediated (insecure pattern). If the anxiety is associated with a cognitive pathway, then disruptions to thinking and perception occur. Upon examination, these patients are frequently suffering from disorganized attachments and unresolved from abuse.

A final example of our approach is presented as an annotated, edited text of a successful 9.5 hours of AB/ISTDP. The process begins with the patient stating their problem and their goal. The author begins by probing the affectively charged areas where the background of the story is told. The patient inevitability begin to defend against the emergence of their traumatized feelings with either defense or superego (negative treatment towards self.) The author next clarifies defenses and discourages the patient from using defenses. Anxiety is mobilized and its pathway is recognized. The patient and author-therapist work hard to overcome the resistance until the traumatized feelings are fully felt and processed by the dyad. The traumatizing other is addressed in a secure coherent way with their role in the trauma. The traumatizing other is symbolically buried and sent on their way. Guilt is felt over whatever aggression is fantasized and the patient learns to compassionately accept their destructive and rageful feelings as part of their historical past. The patient discovers the multigenerational nature of their attachment trauma. As defenses disappear insight (cause and effect) appears and a new calm and somber affect appears. This is reflected back by the therapist and both are in "core state." The relationship complexity between the patient and therapist grow and this facilitates more and deeper explorations into the patients unconscious. In Table 3 the dominant hemisphere associated with the process is noted. I ask the reader to refer to Figure 1 again and to see how this is a dyadic process where feelings are being sent and received via right hemisphere channels and intervention is created and sent by a largely left hemisphere process. The more comfortable the therapist is with switching modes from right to left to right, the smoother the therapy progresses.

Table 3. The Therapeutic Sequence of AB/ISTDP

Therapeutic Sequence	*Dominant Hemisphere*
• Problem telling	Left
• Context or Memory	Left
• Defenses or PSE Present	Right
• Intervention	Both
• PSE and/Defenses go away	Both
• Anxiety emerges	Right
• Anxiety is recognized	Left
• Anxiety overcome	Right
• Unconscious Affect emerges	Right
• Abreaction (Rage, Grief, Guilt,)	Right
• Trauma repaired	Both
• Insight emerges	Synchronization
• Affective relatedness increases	Synchronization ++

(PSE = Punitive Superego)

The Man Who Had to Hang His Head

The patient is a twice-married sixty-three-year-old professional who looks his age. He is of slight stature and has a scholarly look. The patients' areas of disturbance are continuous anxiety, aggravated in performance situations, and low self-esteem, with self-accusations of being a fraud. He has moderate OCD, and undoes his fears with rituals and magical thinking. He avoids intimacy with everyone. He feels that all men are his rivals and believes that this fear began with his father's rejection of him as a child. He says that his father was a kosher butcher, whom he observed cutting the throats of animals. He says his father put him down, made him the butt of jokes, and humiliated him. The psychotherapist pressures the patient to experience his feelings towards his father. The patient becomes resistant, argumentative, and then passive.

We enter eighty minutes into the session when the right hemisphere begins to reveal its presence with imagery.

P: Two images come to mind when you talk about that.
T: mmmhmm
P: both of which are directly physical . . .
T: mmhmm
P I would have cut his beard off.
T: With scissors or a knife?
P: I don't know, probably with a knife.
T: OK.
P: And, the other one is that he used to walk a lot . . . arrogantly showing his body, I would pull his underwear down. His underwear . . . I have never thought about that before.

The session continues after a short break. The patient notes that whenever he visualizes confronting his father, he feels fear and anxiety. We are two hours and twenty minutes into this session.

T: And why does your anxiety go up?
P: the retaliation . . . the fear of retaliation
T: Excellent. "I am afraid my father will kill me. If I stand up for myself, I am afraid he will cut my throat like he did the ox, or the cow, or like he cut."
P: Absolutely, absolutely
T: I'm seeing feeling in you. You don't understand what you have been dealing with. To me, that is a very moving insight and I hope that you will feel your full feeling . . . with respect.
P: Huh?
T: With respect for what you feel. What is the feeling that you feel? The emotion that feel, about having lived like that . . .
P: (sighs)
T: Feel it.
P: What a waste, what a pain.
T: What's the feeling? Empathy isn't it?
P: Empathy, empathy really empathy is . . .
T: Very different
P: Soulness.
T: So from this place inside of you, if you let this side of you become the

most dominant side of you, the most powerful side of you, what would you like to say to yourself? What would your advice be to you?

P: Enough, enough, enough putting your neck down (audible sobbing).

T: To be killed like an animal.

P: (sobbing)

T: Stay . . . stay with your empathy, don't withhold empathy from yourself. OK?

P: Uh, I hope nobody hears me . . . stupid comment.

T: Why is it a stupid comment? It's a putdown isn't it?

P: Yeah

T: it's like your pain, your sadness, for what you suffered is . . .

P: . . . lack of, you know . . .

T: but it is the put down side of you.

P: that is the put down side, the defensive side.

T: Of course.

P: The defensive side.

T: Sure. The side to keep a low profile, you see?

P: Yeah, absolute yes. Yep, yep. That's the side.

T: That lived in so much terror of his father that he couldn't express himself, he, you couldn't assert yourself. You understand that? You feel like every time you assert yourself you have to lay your head down to have your throat cut.

P: Absolutely. It's like I guess if I cut my head, in fact, you know, if I bring my head down it won't be cut. That's exactly it.

T: You have to show submission.

P: Yes, that's exactly, I feel like I am a dog.

T: You feel pain about that, about having to live like that. No human being should . . .

P: I believe you. It's is my secret and nobody knows that. You may know it, but nobody knows it.

T: So how do you feel about the fact that we know it?

P: What?

T: How do you feel about the fact that we know it?

P: Well, I am going to say that I love you for hearing me (audible sobbing).

T: Stay with the love.

P: But then I don't know that I deserve that.

T: (loudly) abababababa—what's that? Catch it.

P: Because it was the anticipation of you kicking my ass and saying "aw, come on, get off it."

T: Do you see how you project your father onto me?

P: Yes, yes.

T: He comes between you and me?

P: Yes.

T: He comes between you and everybody.

P: Yes, absolutely right.

T: So your wife will cut your throat, your friends will cut your throat, anybody you stand up to, even with me, you were standing up for your loving feeling towards me, and you treated yourself like you never deserve to feel it, feel that for me.

P: Yes, absolutely. Right, right.

Accessing his right hemisphere allowed him to see cause and effect, his fear of his father caused him to be submissive and distant. He felt deep compassion for self and close to me but projected his castrating superego into me to attempt to sabotage our connection.

Session 2. The patient returns the next day. He begins the session by recalling that his mother taught him to be afraid of other men. The psychotherapist tells him that he has a choice between continued loyalty to this self-destructive system or freedom from it. The patient reacts with confusion, intellectualization, and then defiance. We are forty-five minutes into the second session.

T: What are your feelings toward me when I say that to you?

P: (hem and haw)

T: Did you have a feeling towards me or not?

P: What do you mean do I have a feeling towards you?

T: Do you have a feeling towards me?

P: I just told you.

T: No you are not, you are being passive.

P: The feeling that you are pushing me (with tension in voice)

T: Not "THAT" why do you have to add "that"?

P: (Chuckles) I feel—

T: What is the feeling, YEAH? I want to know your feeling.

P: I feel you are pushing me (irritated)

T: Now it's "you're pushing me" (with mild irony)

P: wh . . . wha . . . wha . . .

T: Stop with all the linguistic gymnastics

P: (Shows helplessness)

T: What is the feeling you are experiencing towards me? Honest man, direct man. Overcome what your mother told you.

P: I'm doing it (defiantly)

T: I'm waiting, what is the feeling . . . in your body towards me? I am mobilizing, by my behavior a lot of feelings toward me, aren't I? Aren't you having a lot of feelings at me? You have tension in your body. What's making you tense? Own your own feeling!

P: The feeling that I'm not satisfying you.

T: Oh, you go passive, you go submissive (with irony in voice) You do the same behavior, yet you expect a different result. You want to communicate your feeling to me, or not?

P: I'm doing it. (Turns head away.)

T: No you're not—that is absolutely a distortion.

P: The only thing I have now is the image of me grabbing you by the neck (makes strangling motion.)

T: Stay with that. Do not hold back.

P: (Angrily) It's like . . . I have no way to escape.

T: Feel the rage. Don't talk about it, feel it. Describe yourself strangling me, grabbing me by the neck, instead of pushing it down. Encourage yourself to feel it . . . that desire to strangle me.

P: I can't. (Becomes anxious and squirms in chair)

T: Why do you want to go backwards? That's the self-destructive, self-sabotaging, undermining side of you. You break through to the point of imagining killing me, and then you back off, and you won't let yourself enjoy it. Will you let yourself enjoy it for a moment? Did you feel powerful for a second, when you imagined choking me?

P: It was too brief, it was just an image—a fleeting image.

T: Well go back to it.

P: It's gone.

T: (Gently) Go back to it.

P: If I see you as my father, I feel rage. You know something? You look a little like him.

T: And describe?

P: I would push you . . . him, out of the way. I would grab him and get him out of my way.

T: That's a certain degree of your rage. But face the full extent of your rage. You have extensive rage.

P: I don't know if I'm ever capable of feeling the fullest extent of my rage.

T: Now you take a helpless position and you remain loyal to them (the super ego.) Do you want to be loyal to the self-destructive system, to deny your rage—to be passive in the face of your rage? Is that what you want to do? Or do you want to face the full extent of your rage? It's your choice. Do you want to keep hiding your rage—living life like a submissive dog?

P: No, I don't (strongly).

T: So tell me about the rage that's inside the dog . . . if he doesn't cower when he is enraged.

P: You remind me of something. I had a terrible fear as a 3 or 4 year old kid, of dogs. And I think I identified my father as a biting dog.

T: Let's not use projection. You be the biting dog.

P: I'm the fighting dog.

T: Don't project the dog into your father. You be the dog.

P: Then if I'm the dog, I would grab (smacks his lower leg) and go to his throat, and I would be tenacious, and there would be no end to it. The end would be death.

T: Just feel it. The teeth are in your father's neck? Powerful jaws?

After stomping on his father's neck, he guiltily thinks of murdering his mother to gain his freedom. He says "I'd be like Cain, running to the end of the earth." Dr. Neborsky encourages him to speak to her corpse. He is resistant to holding her responsible for manipulating him. He defends her as being sick. But he begins to see that she pulled him into her anxious world and made it impossible for him to leave her in her pain. We are now ninety minutes into the session.

P: Yes. It breaks his neck. All the blood, I guess. All the blood that I've seen flying from chickens would . . . enormous amount of blood.

P: I couldn't walk away.

T: (nods) Tell her.

P: (sighs)

T: Face the truth, it's painful.

P: I have the right to be enraged. She created a miserable life for me (crying). She created a miserable life for me. I was frightened . . . I don't remember a day of not being frightened . . . whether to tell my brother I was doing well in school or whether to go out to the street—frightened of disobeying her. And all this was woven with a great tapestry of love—"You're so special." But she created . . . she castrated me. Maybe she did it. I had thought my father did it.

T: No, she did it. But more specifically, *you did it,* rather than facing your rage at her. And I want to congratulate you for reclaiming your right to your rage.

P: No. She did it. My sympathy for her . . . let me just say to you (points finger at therapist) you're really wonderful. Really. You started saying empathy for myself, why not empathy for this woman?

T: We'll get to that in Part 2. Let's stay with Part 1.

P: OK.

T: You said something about your feelings toward me.

P: You're not, you're not . . . you're doing it for me. You are not doing it for yourself.

After a break, Dr. Neborsky asks the patient to visualize burying his dead mother. At first he is horrified at the thought of touching her, but then he imagines wrapping her in white sheets.

T: What do you do next?

P: Just cry.

T: Cry as long as you want to.

P: (Laughs softly) It's a good way that we part . . . it's a good way that you're dead. I have to remember that you're dead.

T: "I'm not your husband; I've never been your husband."

P: "You treated me like I was better than your husband."

T: "You made me feel like I was better than your husband and that was WRONG"—hold her responsible.

P: Why did you participate in that surreptitious, corruptive game?

T: "I don't want to be your husband . . ." (thirty-second silence) Tell her who she belonged to.

P: My father (laughter). Why don't you accept that I'm just a little child. I can't deliver all that you want me to deliver. You've ruined my life to this point but I won't let you continue to ruin it. In the few years I have left I won't let you ruin it. That's it, rest in peace. (Tearfully recites Kaddish-the Hebrew prayer for the dead.)

T: Feel your grief for your beloved mother. She's only your mother.

P: I love you but leave me alone. I have to be out of that crazy world that you created.

Session 3. The patient returns the next day. He says that whenever he feels an aggressive impulse, he feels guilty. The therapist notes that he allows his conscience to punish him for his fantasies as if they were his actions.

P: Listen, in a court of law, the prosecutor will say "you wish this, you wish this, you wish this, and the prosecutor says if you had the opportunity to stab in the back—without being identified you might being doing it. You haven't quite yet done it . . . but

T: Is the prosecutor on your side?

P: No, he's not!

T: Oh, are you entitled to a defense attorney?

P: Ummm. Oh . . . that's an interesting one (laughs). Oh I see what you are saying.

The patient feels he has found an ally within himself to protect against his punitive super-ego. He remembers how his mother gave him the job of taking care of her emotional needs. He cannot identify the feelings that memory evokes in him. Dr. Neborsky says that his choice is to side either with the crippled part of himself, or the healthy part, and to be free to feel whatever comes up. He begins to process his grief and anger toward his mother but cripples his emotions with anxiety and tension in his chest. The therapist confronts this. We are sixty minutes into this third session and in hour seven of the therapy.

T: Tell your mother of your sadness. Don't put on this false, happy, well-adjusted golden child.

P: Get off my back. Go, let me stay. Go, let me play. Prepare the breakfast. Don't compare me to my brother. Don't tell me I shouldn't complain.

Don't tell me how lucky I am. Don't tell me how reasonable I am, because then I can't (sighing) when I have fears I'm supposed to be the perfect guy.

T: "I will not ever again hide my feelings from you in order to protect you, mother."

P: I will not hide my feelings to protect you. I have to go on with my life. You will have to deal with your own problems. I can't cut my balls for you. (Sighing.) You have to face your own fears. I won't kill you when I tell you that. You won't die and I'm angry at you for putting me through it, for emasculating me. For making me into a hostile, frightened . . .

T: For redirecting my anger away from you, towards everybody else.

P: For redirecting my anger which I should have done to you and now I have felt that my whole world is the enemy, when you are my enemy—you are my enemy. You know, she WAS my enemy. If it weren't for these games, these incentives, unrealistic competition that you seem to encourage between my brother and my father, I would have been happy; I would have had a chance. I paid only to think that you'll give me what I can't take from the world, but you couldn't give it to me. You really couldn't and I didn't turn to the world to get it, and I want to the world. You couldn't give it to me, it was false. You know something, I've paid all this price with relationships so the woman would choose me . . . it was false. I never got it. I never got it! Al I got is the flip side, the race to get rid of everybody else, which was supposed to deliver her, but she really delivered very little.

The patient admits to long-standing hatred for his mother. The therapist asks him to look at what that hatred feels like and what it wants to do. The patient then experiences an impulse to strangle his mother. He visualizes the impulse and begins to resist by shutting down and becoming defiant and intellectual. The psychotherapist confronts his resistance and the patient is given a choice to face his feelings or not. A wave of unconscious guilt passes through his psyche. We return to the interview one hour and twenty minutes into it, as the patient visualizes kissing his mother's murdered corpse.

T: Tell me about the kiss. Feel the kiss.

P: Which I was afraid to do as a child. I kiss her and I would tell her "You go your way, I have to go my way, it will be better this way." (sobbing)

T: Mourn your mother.

P: You meant well, but you couldn't do it.

T: "You created these murderous feelings in me and I have been prosecuting myself as though I were a criminal because I couldn't face the full extent of my murderous rage toward you, mother. I couldn't do it until now."

P: And I couldn't. And I felt that your love was conditional upon my getting rid of other men. This was the insidious thing. It was conditional upon this. I walked around trying to kill the men in the world, to win you.

T: To make her happy.

P: To make her happy so she could love me. Yes, yes, that was the trade-off, that was the legacy (Begins rubbing his neck) It's over, it's over.

The patient contrasts his experience of these three ISTDP sessions with his twenty years of psychoanalysis.

P: I understood a lot of it, but I did not understand the need to separate and to be proactive about it. I was talking with somebody yesterday and what is so unique and refreshing about it is what you said in the first meeting with me, "Is this the healthy part or the sick part?" That is very important for me. Because in the other therapy it was like a continuum, the lines are not drawn very clearly to separate them, label and make you aware. Not to give in to the unhealthy part. That was an eye opener. For me it was very very important.

T: Define the healthy part?

P: The healthy part is the part that wants to be free, that wants to walk straight . . .

T: And wants to explore and investigate his feelings.

P: I wouldn't have added those terms.

T: The part that wants to investigate his rage, his grief, his sexual feelings.

P: I wouldn't have added grief. I would always shut myself off and would walk away, and it is a self-destructive part of my defenses. This is really remarkable, I am counting on it. I am feeling like I am on a threshold. I really have to tell you (leans forward, touches the leg of the therapist), I have to tell you very positive, but very profound. It's not like, "Gee, I'm a new man"; it is very somber, but very liberating—like I've gotten the key.

Session 4. The patient returns five days later for his termination session. He is now able to feel rage towards his mother without resistance. He visualizes killing her by cutting off her head with a sword. He visualizes burying her, and, once more, kissing her dead body.

P: I guess I will have to kiss her good-bye.

T: Describe the kiss.

P: I would hold her and kiss her, which reminds me of when I was a kid. She would grab me to kiss me and I was afraid, because I thought she would seduce me. But I'm not afraid anymore. I didn't have the comfort of a mother, any real comfort, any care of a mother, because she claimed she was ill. She couldn't do, she couldn't get out of bed.

T: Tell her.

P: You couldn't prepare meals, you couldn't prepare the house, you continuously frightened us that you would have a heart attack. We couldn't disagree with you because you would get agitated and have a heart attack. You surrounded us with unreal dangers, a frightening world, frightening events that would happen—it was a nightmare, Dr. Neborsky, it was a nightmare. (yells) IT WAS A NIGHTMARE. (sobs) IT WAS A NIGHTMARE and it continues . . . (sobbing)

T: Face your grief and face your rage.

P: She caused it, she caused it. But why do I fall back to sympathy for myself, for the nightmare? I guess I deserve the sympathy, I deserve it. (sobbing) God knows I deserve it.

T: Yes you do.

P: I have never cried like this, it was a nightmare from the moment I got up to the moment I went to sleep, I was frightened, and the bed-wetting. The enemies, the evil eye, and her sickness. OH MY GOD, I had no life. No life. And I barely managed to maintain this façade. I've got to change. You should have looked after me. THAT'S IT . . . You didn't look after me. You looked after your own. I'm now strong enough to look into my anger against you, mother. I am strong enough to walk away from you. I am strong enough to say good-bye to you. I'm strong enough to know you are buried and I can go on with my life. Yes, you are out of my life. I will not do it again.

T: Do what again?

P: Allow myself to speak for you and to subjugate me. If I don't allow myself, then I won't allow other people. But I have been doing it, I have been doing it and I've been doing it, not realizing that I've been speaking your voice. But you have no voice anymore . . . you have no voice. You are just a body, just a corpse.

T: "I choose to bury you."

P: And now you are buried. I choose to bury you, so I don't have to have you on my arm, back of my head, you're gone. Bye bye.

The psychotherapist interprets that he rejected his father because his mother unconsciously encouraged it.

T: Your father did let you down, but at the same time, I would sense that you didn't give him a chance, either.

P: That's true. Yes, yes, it was a mutual non-recognition of each other. I treated him in some way, as an imposter, and that's sad—because of my mother. He was very aloof and insecure and maybe was challenged by me in some ways.

T: In many ways, your mother set you up to be the husband and him to be the outsider.

P: You mean she had the INTENTION to separate us? You're not confident in that. Why do you say that?

She did it, she shouldn't have done it, but I don't know that she WANTED me separated from my father . . . Why? (appears stunned) (silence.)

Yes. There is no shred of doubt about it. The Interpretation. NO shred of doubt. It makes me sad again.

T: Let me hear the words between you and your mother.

P: I'm going away now. I'm leaving you behind. I have to go away. But even if you were alive, I would have been away from you now. I've severed the ties. I've cut the rope. I now understand how you have used me, have acted the opposite of a mother. You have made me insecure, you have frightened me, you have turned me into what I have feared, which was a beast . . . worse than a beast. You made me competitive, hateful of other men, and insecure with women. And that has ended. I've seen through it. I've seen that it was all out of your needs. The world is not like that.

Men are not my rivals. My father was not my rival, because you were not my wife. You were never going to be my wife. No he was not, and I projected on him for a long time.

T: Yeah.

As a way of deconstructing his OCD, he remarks on the world of fear and superstition his mother surrounded him with, "from morning till night." We are eighty-five minutes into this termination session, and nine hours into treatment.

P: To some extent it was a perversion of reality. The reality was not reassuring.

T: Amplification, all danger was amplified.

P: And, in a scary way, potentially under your control, if only you carried garlic and salt to ward off the evil eye. If only you don't go to the street . . . If only you don't think about going to sleep, you fall asleep.

And as a result of it, I, all my life, tried to deal with the world . . . Now I'm getting uptight because I'm controlling the fear with . . .

T: Through magic.

P: With magic or with your body. The body was perverted, instead of reassuring. Oh my God! It's as I talk about it, I just realized for the first time I have more sympathy for the world I've lived in. It's a world of horrors. From the moment you get up, there is nothing reassuring. It wasn't: so if you're afraid about hunger—but you have love and protection. It's a world of running away and manipulation—hiding . . . say good-bye to that.

After a five-minute break, the patient says that his psychoanalyst never explored his relationship with his mother in any depth. He expresses gratitude for the clarity he has now.

P: He talked about that she wasn't caring for me, he didn't put it together, to stay on it. That is news to me after 20 years. You can see I have a lot of insights, which if you do it long enough, you become introspective. But I didn't see that.

T: I noticed a rise of emotion towards me.

P: I'm sad that I'm going away, but that's life. I have to go away. I have to work on it. I have to remember and I have to fight it.

T: Emotions toward me.

P: Which is quite different from when I came in. I'm in shock. I didn't get to the point of seeing my mother critically, or feeling my rage, or even thinking that I was entitled to it. And as a result of that, she was always benevolent, and enticing. She had an enticing side to her. For a child, it was very intoxicating. "I'm going to make you better than your father." That was the payoff for which I gave up my will. I gave up any resistance. I went beyond it for the little favors. She created an idealized image of me and I created an idealized image of her, and we were trading.

T: That's correct.

P: And this is a very corrupting, very sinister, destructive—it sucks you in, gratifying at a certain level. In the system, the rest of the world was your enemies . . . and I see it now. I reject it. I've seen it already with my life, even after just three days here. What I'm doing to her is unfair . . . trying to suck her into that game.

T: Oh, you are doing to her, what your mother did to you.

P: Yeah, trying to suck her into that game. "If you would just understand me, I wouldn't have to express my wishes, and all the other things that go with it." I created a problem with my wife, with sex and other things. Here's the other thing: my mother—my wife, I was going to say—continuously always tested me.

So, you have to perform. She couldn't just confer it, and it's done, so I am sucked in, into this rivalrous activity . . . and I'm always afraid that I will fail . . . in that enticing, collusive, seductive relationship that I am recognizing and rejecting. So I have a lot to do.

T: So there is going to be a lot of change in the relationship with your wife, as you set her free.

P: ABSOLUTELY. And I've seen it already . . . it's very nice. I've seen it with her, and I've seen it with men. I've seen the impact already. It's the right solution for me. It feels terrific. I have to thank you.

Despite twenty years of psychoanalysis, this patient still carried within himself a punitive superego and used highly maladaptive defense. Beneath this self-punitive and defensive structure lay his unresolved attachment trauma. It was concealed by a prolonged unconscious idealization of his mother. He continued to enact the script which his histrionic, seductive and superstitious mother played out with him in their attachment to each other. She mandated that he always be "the best" in order to ward off danger—if he was she rewarded him with her exclusive love. We see multiple possible unresolved attachment traumas. His actual non idealized experience was that his mother was "unloving" (narcissistic, somatic, manipulative), "involving/reversing" (son replacing father as idealized love object) and used "pressure to achieve" on him in order to satisfy her needs. These traumas created a severely disturbed oedipal relationship with his father resulting in both a symptom and character neurosis. Both of these malignant structures were deconstructed in this therapy. By my measures, the patient left therapy a changed man. Healthy self-assertion replaced fearful submission. His genuine longings for intimacy with his wife and male friends became actualized. His anxiety disappeared and his OCD normalized.

Two people—patient and therapist come together in a therapeutic venture. The therapist listens and absorbs historical and dynamic information that activates the mind of the therapist. The therapist with ISTDP technique can access the patient's unconscious in a remarkably short period of time by following the sequence of interventions invented by Davanloo and elaborated by Malan. If the dyad can overcome the constraints placed against feeling traumatically based emotion, rapid and long lasting change can and does occur. Deeply felt long lasting emotional insights sustain the patient and reinforce the changes made during the psychotherapy. Mastery of this process is a lifelong effort which has endless frustrations as well as endless rewards. The authors thank their teachers, patients and students for their role in developing their understanding of the unconscious mind and how access it in order to transform trauma to triumph.

BIBLIOGRAPHY

Ainsworth, M.D.S., Blehar, M.C. Waters, E., & Wall, S. (1978). *Patterns of attachment: A psychologic study of the Strange Situation.* Hillsdale, NJ: Ehrbaum.

Beebe, B., Jaffe, J. & Lachman, (1994). A dyadic systems model of mother-infant mutual regulation: Implications for the origins of representations and therapeutic interactions. *Psychoanalytic Psychologist* 1994 14: 27–33.

Beebe, B. & Lachman, (2002). *Infant Research and Adult Treatment.* Hillsdale, NJ: Analytic Press.

Davanloo, H. (1990). Clinical Manifestations of Superego Pathology. *Unlocking the Unconscious.* Chichester: Wiley.

Freud, S. (1900/1958) Sexuality in the aetiology of the neuroses *SE: III*: pp 259–285 London.

Lyons-Ruth, K. (2002) *Dissociation and the Parent-Infant Dialogue: A longitudinal perspective from attachment research. J American Psychoanalytic Assn 51*:3, 883–911.

Leichsenring, F, Rabung, S, Leibing,. (2004). The Efficacy of Short-Term Dynamic Psychotherapy in Specific Psychiatric Disorders: A Meta-analysis. *Arch Gen Psychiatry. 61*:1208–1216.

Malan, D. (2001)The Road Ahead. in Solomon, M., Neborsky, R.J., et al. *Short-Term Therapy for Long-Term Change.* New York: WW Norton & Co.

Malan, D. and Coughlin, P. (2007) *Lives Transformed.* Karnac: London.

Main, M. and Goldwin, R (1998) *Adult attachment scoring and classification system.* Unpublished scoring manual v. 6.3, UC Berkeley.

Main, M. and Hesse, E. (1990). Parents' unresolved traumatic experiences are related to infant disorganized attachment status: Is frightened parental behavior the linking mechanism? In M.T. Greenberg, D. Chicchetti & E. M. Cummings (Eds.), *Attachment in the preschool years: theory, research, and intervention,* (pp 161–182). Chicago: University of Chicago Press.

Neborsky, R.J. (2003). Healing Trauma: an affect experiencing attachment theory model for comprehensive treatment of trauma. In Solomon, M Siegel, D (ed.) *Healing Trauma,* New York: WW. Norton & Co.

Neborsky, R.J. (2003) Shame and Guilt from a Developmental Neuroscience Perspective: Implications for Technique in Intensive Short-Term Dynamic Psychotherapy. Part I. *Ad Hoc Bulletin of Short-term Dynamic Psychotherapy* 7 (1), 54–75.

Neborsky, R.J. (2004) Recognizing and working with an Oedipal Focus in ISTDP. Part I. and II *Ad Hoc Bulletin of Short-term Dynamic Psychotherapy* 8 (1, 2), 29–44.

Neborsky, R.J. (2001) Changing the Love Imprint. in Solomon, M., Neborsky, R.J., et al. *Short-Term Therapy for Long-Term Change.* New York: WW Norton & Co.

Neborsky, (2004b) Can attachment status be predicted from a recorded clinical interview? Study in Progress. UCSD School of Medicine Human Subjects Project 030445.

Pearson, J.L. Cohn, D.A., Cowan, P.A. & Cowan, P.C. (1994) Earned and continuous security in adult attachment: relation to depressive symptomatology and parenting style. *Development and Psychopathology, 6,* 259–373.

Shore, A.N. (1996) The experience-dependent maturation of a regulatory system in the orbital prefrontal cortex and the development of psychopathology. *Development and Psychopathology, 8,* 59–87.

Shore, A.N. (2002) Dysregulation of the right brain: a fundamental mechanism of traumatic attachment and the pathogenesis of post-traumatic stress disorder. *Australian and New Zealand Journal of Psychiatry;* 36:9–30.

Sroufe, L.A., Engeland, B., & Krentger, T. (1990). The fate of early experience following developmental change: Longitudinal approaches to individual adaptation in childhood. *Child Development, 54,* 1615–1627.

Journal of Clinical Psychology: In Session, Vol. 62 (5) 523–538. May 2006.

Identifying and Overcoming the Punitive Superego in Short-term Dynamic Psychotherapy

The Man with a Pain in His Chest

WITH EMANUEL PELUSO, MFT

In this article the authors review the historical roots of the concept of the superego from an analytical perspective. They articulate specific criterion for diagnosing a punitive superego and outline a system for de-identifying patients from their punitive superego part. They discuss the different points of view about the origin of the punitive superego and the importance of making the unconscious feelings of guilt, conscious as early in therapy as possible. An illustrative clinical case is summarized and annotated with vignettes following a modified central dynamic sequence in a fifteen-hour block therapy case with good clinical results. Finally the authors suggest a metaphor for the metapsychology of clinical cure from Greek Mythology.

Freud introduced the term superego (Über-ich) in 1923, but he had been forming his concept of it for years, drawing his ideas from mythology, his insight with patients, and especially his self-analysis, in which he first glimpsed the primary source of the superego's development, the Oedipal complex. The Oedipal myth, Freud wrote, "seizes on a compulsion which everyone recognizes because he feels its existence within himself." (Freud, 1897) The universality of this "compulsion" leads to the conclusion that it is either genetic, or stems from a common historical event.

It was the latter possibility that interested Freud. In *Totem and Taboo* (Freud 1912), he speculated that prehistorical society organized itself into patriarchal groups, with one dominant male hording the females. As his male progeny matured, each boy was banished to prevent him from one day challenging his father's rule. But some of these young men eventually banded together, killed their father, and gained access to the females, who were, of course, their own mothers. But after the murder, the men were filled with grief and guilt, and with the dawning possibility that their own sons would one day repeat their act against themselves. They therefore declared that patricide "was not allowed, and (they) renounced the fruits of their deed by denying themselves the liberated (mothers). (Freud, 1912, p 185)

This injunction became an unconscious part of the human psyche, but the "compulsion"—fraught with desire, guilt and grief—still persisted in that same psyche. In a sense, then, Freud came to see that the tragedy of the patricidal myth was still being acted out in our own era—bloodlessly to be sure—within each child's intrapsychic drama of inferred paternal castration and imagined patricide. With the resolution of this "Oedipal complex," Freud theorized, the maturing child introjected the values of his/her "parental agency" (Freud, 1933) and, by implication, the mores of the social group, into a differentiated structure within the ego, the superego (Freud, 1923; 1940). Of particular importance in this theory is Freud's statement that "a child's superego is in fact constructed on the model not of its parents, but of its parents' superego; the contents which fill it are the same and it becomes the vehicle of tradition[s] . . . which have propagated themselves in this manner from generation to generation." (Freud, 1933, S.E. XXII, p. 67)

As Freud sought to understand the negative therapeutic reactions in his patients, he came to see the superego as a potentially malevolent force, which causes the patient to blindly prefer continued distress to cure. Freud had seen that a tyrannical superego, in effect, made demands that were so "powerful and so relentless that the ego may be paralyzed. (Freud, 1940, pp. 172–173)." It became, in one writer's vivid phrasing, an "insatiable tyrant . . . (which) . . . under the mask of a concern with social peace and union, carries on a ceaseless aggression to no purpose save that of the enhancement of its own power, inflicts punishment for no act committed but only for a thought denied, and, so far from being appeased by acquiescence in its demands, actually increases its severity in the degree that is obeyed." (Trilling, 1971)

Davanloo agreed with Freud that as long as the therapy was under the domination of this punitive force—that is, the patient's "need for punishment" (Freud, 1924)—therapeutic change would be ineffective, superficial, and attenuated. Freud acknowledged that the mechanism of guilt remained invisible to his patient ". . . as far as the patient is concerned this sense of guilt is dumb; it does not tell him he is guilty; he does not feel guilty, he feels ill. This sense of guilt expresses itself only as a resistance to recovery which is extremely difficult to overcome" (Freud, 1923, The Ego and the Id). Davanloo sought a way to quickly neutralize, not only the power of the superego, but also to make its crippling effect apparent in the therapeutic session. Davanloo had a subset of patients who suffered from severe emotional symptoms (some percent of which somatized as well), who had chronic problems with closeness and intimacy, and who habitually sabotaged their opportunities in life. Davanloo discovered that when he explicitly acquainted these patients with their "punitive" superegos, exposed its pathogenic origin, and demonstrated how it was operating in the here-and-now *in their first evaluation* their progress in treatment accelerated. He found, too, that this same class of patients suffered attachment disruptions in their early childhood, ranging from abandonment to abuse, over-protection and over-control and concluded that this disruption, contrary to psychoanalytic theory, was central to the pathologic development of their punitive psychic structure.

In Davanloo's opinion, Freud's view of the superego's development, based solely on the resolution of the Oedipal complex, was "narrow" and outdated, and thought it "surely . . . should be assigned to the historical museum" (Davanloo, 1990, p. 190). Davanloo suggested, for example, that a father's sadism might be a more obvious explanation of his child's murderous impulses; as could very early, pre-Oedipal rage at being displaced by a sibling.

We (Neborsky, 2001), like Davanloo, in our working schema, view the development of an unhealthy superego as primarily the result of early broken bonds of attunement, compassion and empathy. These forms of attachment traumas then cause the child to experience reactive aggression against that parent along with commensurate fears of retaliation. When these traumas occur early in development and are repetitive, devastating psychic damage is often the result. Such people present in our practices as adults who are overly critical and neglectful of themselves, who often place and keep themselves in situations where they are victimized, and who avoid closeness or intimacy with others.

On the other hand, the development of a healthy and loving superego occurs when the bond of attunement, compassion and empathy are maintained. This creates an internalized flexible, constructive, and loving object relationship with the self. The healthy superego has the following characteristics or functions: It realistically praises, supports, values and encourages knowing ones feelings; it encourages autonomy and free choice; it empathizes with disappointment and failure, and takes constructive action in the face of failure; it supports empathy and consideration for the rights of others which conflict with freedom of the self. Patients with such a history present with low resistance and their grief and guilt are readily accessible.

A punitive superego operates more rigidly and prevents the therapist and patient from forming a healthy alliance. It enforces its imperatives through fear or through seduction; it offers "love" (*i.e.*, the illusion of secure attachment) to the ego through obedience to an authoritarian structure or through loyalty to a belief system; it maintains an inflexible, destructive, and unloving object relationship with the ego which it scolds and shames when disobeyed; it discourages knowing one's feelings; it encourages repression; it demands loyalty for its love; and, by ignoring emotions and psychological insight, it prevents learning from failing strategies.

Changing Punitive Superegos

Freud reportedly became pessimistic about psychoanalysis's ability to alter the punitive superego's hold on the psyche (Freud, 1926). He saw its resistance as "the most powerful factor and the one most dreaded by us," and one he was forced to "bow to the superiority" of because "even to exert a psychical influence on simple masochism is a severe strain tax on our powers" (Freud, 1937). Davanloo's approach, in contrast, is more optimistic. Josette ten Have-de Labije (2001) has taken this approach one step beyond Davanloo in her version of ISDTP. The patient is encouraged to become an active agent in the deconstruction of his punitive side, and the therapist acts as an external and alternative superego—loving and healthy—until the patient can internalize those qualities. The patient is encouraged to look at himself with love and precision and care, to differentiate this from his punitive/sadistic superego eyes and voice. Additionally, the patient is encouraged to understand that his defenses are in fact his obedience to his internalized punitive, sadistic superego, and that they perpetuate his suffering. He is challenged to relinquish these defenses. Once this milestone is achieved, the new healthy superego is internalized from the therapeutic relationship and becomes installed as a new part of the self.

To build this alliance, the patient is helped to separate the constructive ego part from the punitive super ego part. This is accomplished by 1) drawing the patient's attention to his decision and wish to develop insight into his intimate thoughts, feelings and dynamic processes, 2) by drawing the patient's attention to his automatic refuge to his ego-syntonic defense, 3) by drawing the patient's attention to their self-destructive function, by challenging the patient to relinquish these self-destructive defenses, 4) allowing the patient to feel grief over living under the dominance of these defenses.

The decision to seek therapy is a major act of separation from the punitive superego and the patient is acknowledged by the therapist for their courage in that act. At the same time the patient's habitual and automatic defenses are brought to their awareness. The patient is encouraged to see the way these defensive activities maintain the status quo and cause the sabotage of the process.

Figure 1. shows the model of the psyche which we use in working with patient's with punitive superego's.

As the therapy deepens and moves forward, the superego loses more control over the ego. The patient becomes able to consciously explore his dynamic processes, and to direct his attention to his physical experience of core emotions, their cognitive contents, and their action tendency. Notice in Figure 1 how some aspects of the model are conscious, others are unconscious. As the therapy progresses consciousness becomes more and more the dominant domain.

Figure 1. Dynamic Origin of Punitive Superego and Its Maintenance (ten Have-de Labije and Neborsky)

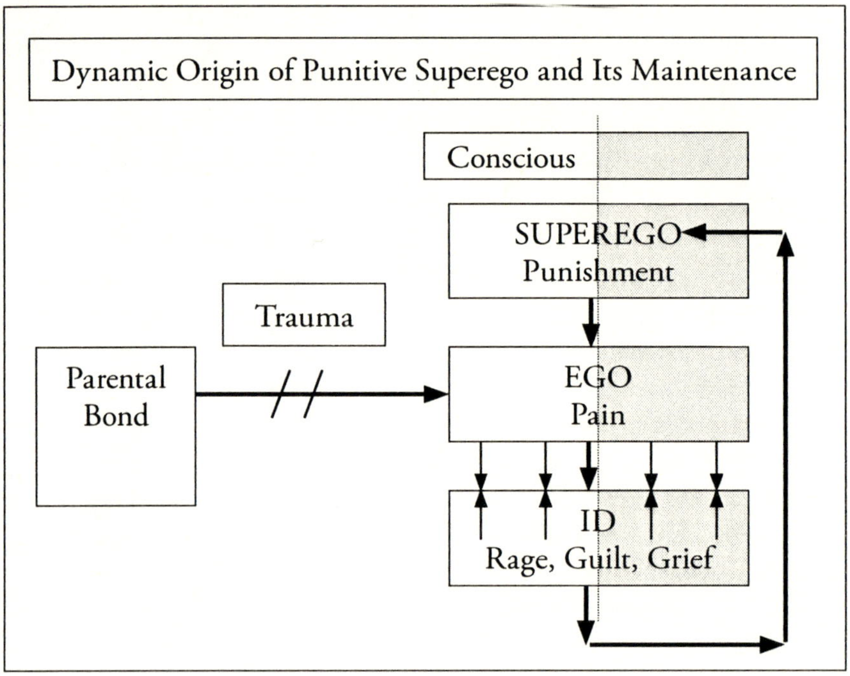

In summary, trauma in the attachment bond—by a parent, for instance—causes the ego pain. This leads to rage and to murderous and sadistic fantasies, followed by guilt over the rage, and grief over the imagined murder. The ego tries to bury these deeds and complex feelings in the id. But forces of de-repression threaten to bring it all back to consciousness, so all is buried into a differentiated part of the ego. But the battle to keep the material from view is exhausting and interminable. Taking a cue from Freud, if we visualize this process in mythic terms, the child kills the parent, buries the corpse, which then rises from the grave as a specter to haunt the perpetrator with punishing, paralyzing suffering. In this way, the mythic cycle is complete. The parent has created in the child the same punitive superego from which the parent itself suffered. This superego then relentlessly punishes the ego with pain. This pain produces even more rage, which is repressed into the id, causing the superego to demand even more suffering. The self is at war with itself and the more identified the self is with this punitive superego, the less able it is to challenge, much less kill it.

The following annotated case shows how one of the authors applied this model to the short-term treatment of a patient with a highly punitive superego. He was treated in 5 consecutive days with 3 hour therapy blocks. Each session largely followed a modification of Davanloo's Central Dynamic Sequence as described by ten Have-de Labije (2001) The vignettes are chosen to demonstrate the elements of this patient's experience that lead to his developing a punitive superego and the way in which it is a) "exposed "and b) deactivated by allowing the ego to feel the complex emotions which were at one time, intolerable.

Case Report: The Man with Pain in his Heart

The patient is a fifty-two-year-old single man who works as a fireman. He was referred to Dr. Neborsky by his EAP counselor who felt that his difficulties were appropriate for Attachment-Based Short-term Dynamic Psychotherapy. The patient has been suffering from low-grade depression with intermittent levels of anxiety which have progressively impaired his health and cognitive performance. He recently complained of chest pain for which he had a physical exam. No medical conditions were found. He also reports breakthroughs of anger and irritability of increasing intensity. He has no alcohol or chemical dependency problems and he is on no medication.

His diagnosis qualifies for dysthymic disorder and atypical anxiety disorder with avoidant personality traits.

The patient reports divorcing his wife eight years ago because of "lack of intimacy" in the relationship. He reports great ease in attracting women but admits that he is himself incapable of maintaining and sustaining a close relationship. He loves his two children, but laments that they are emotionally distant from him. In addition to depression and anxiety with physical and cognitive aspects, he complains of loneliness and feels hopeless about ever finding a woman to whom he could both trust and commit. He recently broke up with a woman whom he loved but could not bring himself to trust.

We will open with a vignette of the patient describing the presenting problem on day one.

Vignette 1

The inquiry explores the patient's difficulties and the patient's initial ability to respond.

T: So let's start again with the areas of disturbance—the things you'd like to get addressed and fixed inside.

P: There are several. Lately, I just haven't been happy, y'know. I'm struggling within relationships. Just, I guess, general unhappiness. I'm angry a lot of the time; I'm impatient . . .

T: I keep asking you about the intensity of the anger. That's seems like something you won't tell me about, y'know.

P: I'm not sure exactly what you mean. Intensity—you mean what I actually do with it?

T: You don't know what I mean by the intensity? How it feels inside?

P: Yeah, it feels bad.

T: Describe it.

P: It's almost that I can't control it, I can't just put it on the backburner.

T: You're again describing how you can handle it, what you can do with it, what you can't do with it, but I'm asking you how it feels inside. And what I'm observing is, you try and tell me, there's seems to be almost a barrier in you—it's not your fault, I'm just telling you—that you can't address you anger with me in a very clear way. Now, what do you feel in your body? What are you noticing inside as we talk about this?

P: Frustration that I can't get it out.

T: Sure. But that makes a lot of sense, doesn't it? If you've got a wall between you and your feeling part, you would be frustrated. That's a natural result of having a wall. So the tension, it seems to me, is pretty clear to you. That's a clear signal, that you can feel that in your body.

P: Mmhm.

T: Where do you feel the tension in your body?

P: I can't really put my finger on it, I guess. Just not relaxed.

T: So you're hitting up against that wall again.

In the inquiry phase the therapist also puts mild pressure on the patient's vague defenses and quickly assessed a power struggle would be useless. The therapist decides to draw the patient's attention to his ego-syntonic defense of ignoring and to encourage the patient to observe.

Vignette 2

Helping the Patient Build An Observing-Ego: Pressure to experience is applied in order to crystallize the character resistance in the transference. Thus the discussion of "the wall" refers to the resistance. We are thirteen minutes into the session.

T: Could you a see a way that would cause you any problems in your life?
P: Mmhm.
T: Like what?
P: Well, if I'm not aware of it, I'm going to react to that feeling and I'm going to vent in negative ways, in anger . . .
T: Till it explodes, kind of? In other words, you'll ignore it, ignore it, ignore it, until you can't handle it anymore and you'll just have an outburst, or you'll act out on it, kind of, to get rid of it.
P: (Nods)
T: Yeah, that's the problem I would see with that. So it seems to me that's the first order of business is for you to break that habit.
P: Mmhm.
T: If that's causing you a problem, you see. Now how long in your life have you been like this? How long have you taken this ignoring position toward your emotional part?
P: Probably my whole life . . .

The patient has observed an ego-syntonic defense—ignoring—and also understands its self-destructive function. The therapist then applies pressure for specificity.

T: But did you think of something specific in your mind that led you to ignore your feeling part? Was there a specific incident from your childhood or relationship that was particularly troubled for you?

P: See, I'm just getting all confused now; my mind's sort of going all over the place; and I'm struggling to focus on something, per se, y'know, it was . . .

T: Wait, wait, please. You just told me you were having a problem so let's not ignore it, right.

The therapist makes the defense of ignoring distress ego-dystonic. This is a major attachment failure and a sign of a punitive superego. Furthermore it is apparent that superego projection is occurring and it will threaten the working alliance. The patient is projecting his punitive superego part onto the therapist and regressing from fear of his retaliation. The therapist immediately begins to clarify and asked the patient to intervene on his own behalf.

P: OK.

T: Wouldn't that be the worst behavior I could engage in were I to ignore it, when you told me you were having a problem? What do you think is causing your confused mental state right now? What do you think is going on inside?

Even though the therapist is talking about "me," he is really modeling a constructive superego and contrasting it to the patient's projected punitive superego.

P: . . . I'm not sure. I want to change it.

T: But I just want to point it out again—"I'm not sure"—that's that kind of habitual, chronic way you have of ignoring and neglecting your emotional part. You tell me you feel bad, and I believe you; I know you're telling me the truth, but you don't tune into the feeling part, you see? This side of you that says—and I'll be a little dramatic here—"Ralph, your feelings are not important; ignore 'em; keep on truckin'; go through life; get money; be successful; that's the important thing here. Don't stop to take a careful inventory of what you're feeling." It's a side of your personality, you see?

The therapist identifies the message from the punitive superego that rules the patient's existence.

P: Mmhm.

T: The part that says that, "If you feel bad, don't tune into the fact that you feel bad; move on to other things."

P: I guess it's something that's been taught to me my whole life. It's never been OK, y'know? You just gotta be strong and push on.

T: And you see that that stance, which I understand why you adopted it—it's very clear to me—but you see, in here, it works against your purposes.

P: Yeah, I understand that.

T: If you want this to be successful—here, with me—you gotta take exactly the opposite stance toward yourself. Which is what you feel is of paramount importance in here—something to be noticed and carefully paid attention to.

P: Yeah.

T: Otherwise, this is going to be a very ineffective week for you.

P: Yeah, I understand that. And I'll do my best, you know.

T: You're able to implement that, in other words.

P: I'm sure hoping I can.

T: Well, let's give it a go, OK?

The patient's commitment to seek therapy is honored (valued) and this is set against his obedience to the avoidant attachment rules that he lives by. A mild challenge is administered to further separate him from his loyalty to his punitive superego.

Vignette 3

Observing ego learns to identify his feelings, defenses, and current psychic dynamic activity. We are twenty-six minutes into the session.

T: So maybe you could tell me a little more specifically about the family trouble that started your problem—why you had to adopt this self-negligent position here: you put your feelings away and build a wall around yourself and just focus on bettering yourself. Where did that start?

P: I imagine that started with my parents. You don't have to be a brain surgeon to figure out what I went through in my childhood; I had a bad childhood, with alcoholic parents. My father was a hard-assed firefighter as well, and he was very mean. He's passed away now; so is my mum. (Sighs.) Yeah, you had to be tough around him.

T: I see.

P: And, y'know, he was very unsupportive. I never felt any love from him; I don't think he was capable of it.

T: I see.

P: I feel sorry for him now, and y'know, I've forgiven him.

T: Mmhm. Now, I'm noticing as we talk about this a rise in your emotional part. Your feeling parts are trying to push themselves up. Are you noticing that too?

P: Nah . . . (sighs).

T: Your speech got a little slower. Your words got more and more carefully expressed. I even noticed some tightness in your chest. Did you notice that as well?

P: No, not really. I think I calmed down a bit.

T: You calmed down a bit. OK.

P: I guess it's probably because . . . Now, I'm feeling that sort of confusion again. Just right now.

T: You are? Good. Not good that you're confused; good that you're noticing it and good that you're telling it. Now, what does that confusion represent to you if we're going to label it?

P: Anxiety. Pressure. I'm feeling pressured to get it all right and clear.

T: So that's another thing you do to yourself, then? In other words, you put pressure on yourself to perform.

P: Oh, without a doubt. Yeah.

T: So that was another one of those things you did to yourself, kind of, make something out of yourself?

P: Mmhm.

T: Did your father put pressure on you, too?

P: Mmhm.

T: He was that kind of father, put pressure on you.

P: Mmhm.

T: OK. And is the mental confusion still with you right now or has it gone back down?

P: It went down a bit.

T: Good. So you see, when you label it as anxiety, I think it helps you lower it.
P: Mmhm. That makes sense.

The patient's ability to observe his emotional processes collapsed under the weight of his anxiety. His anxiety was created by his superego projection into me and in the transference feeling that I was his father and he had to submit and perform for me. This occurs in patients who are identified with their punitive superegos.

Vignette 4

The Observing Ego Improves: The patient experiences a brief sad feeling for himself with the thought that he was never held as a baby. We are thirty-five minutes into the session.

T: And I'm asking you, when you connect to that sad feeling, do you feel better or do you feel worse?
P: (Sighs) I feel, uh, probably more in touch with myself.
T: But I'm asking as you sit here with me, does that being more in touch with yourself, does that feel good to you or does that feel bad to you?
P: I'd take it over the confusion and the anxiousness.
T: Mmhm. Yeah, I would too, every day. So to me that's a positive. Is it to you?
P: Mmhm.
T: OK, so can we make a statement here and you and I agree on it? So, when you're in touch with your feelings, your true feelings, that it's a better thing for you than to be hiding behind a wall of anxiety and confusion.
P: Mmhm.
T: Would you say that to me?
P: It's a better place to be rather than hiding behind a wall of anxiety and confusion. It's better to be in touch with your feelings.

The patient is encouraged to take an active stance against his punitive devaluing, avoidant superego.

Vignette 5

Building an Attentive Ego, Experiencing Compassion for Self: The therapist asks the patient to recall one painful childhood memory. The patient says that he again feels confused.

T: But if you notice that if every time I ask you an emotionally charged question, that's going to bring more true feelings out of you, your anxiety goes up. If you could just see it as a wall. I ask you to tell me one painful memory from your childhood . . .

P: . . . which should be very easy.

The therapist is uncertain as to whether this was a self put-down or cooperation:

T: Well, I'm not sure what you mean by that. I mean, it's obviously going to bring more feelings up. It's not *that* easy. It's a loaded question, isn't it?

P: Yeah.

T: The anxiety goes up, the confusion. The old you would attack you, put you down, make you feel helpless, call him bad names. "Get movin', get on the road, get workin'." You see the pattern?

P: Yes.

T: So what I'm trying to get you to do here with me is notice that rise of anxiety and understand it's because the emotional part of you is getting triggered. And the job for us is to lower your anxiety by bringing these feelings out of you. Does that make sense?

P: Yeah.

T: Do you see how predictable it is for you? How it just happens each time we do it?

P: Mmhm.

T: See, each time we do it, as long you don't go to criticizing yourself for doing it, but you notice it and address it in a kind way. Can you see the importance of that?

P: Totally.

Vignette 6

Helping the Patient Unmask and Identify His Punitive Superego: The patient relates a childhood incident in which his father was furious at him for losing a swimming race. We are fifty minutes into the session.

T: And just as you have that brief memory here, tell me what you notice inside.

P: It didn't really register too much.

T: What didn't register too much? I don't really understand what you mean.

P: Speaking about that incident.

T: See, but how is that possible?

P: Maybe I'm blocking it out.

T: What I'm saying is, the only way that could be possible is you were using some sort of defense mechanism to keep your emotions at bay. The only reason you remember this is because it has a lot of emotions around it, right?

P: And you know, the funny thing is, it's as clear in my head as if it was yesterday.

T: OK. So what do you think you're doing?

P: Blocking.

T: Blocking the emotions.

P: I can't even tell you what it was exactly . . .

T: Now, if we're talking about who's running the session right now: Is the guy who brought you here, and who wanted to address his emotions running the session, or is the part of you that learned how to defend against his emotions, by being a compulsive overachiever, by putting himself down, by ignoring himself and his emotions—is he running the session right now?

P: Probably him.

T: If he runs the session, what's going to be the result of the session?

P: Not much.

T: Same as always. It's just going to reinforce that behavior, see? That's where I need you to step up the plate here. You need to be willing to say no to that side of yourself. Remember, a few minutes ago, you were telling me you were angry at that side of yourself?

P: Mmhm.

T: You felt a real anger?

P: Mmhm.

T: So are you willing to take control of the session?

P: I'd love to. I'm not sure if I know how, but I would love to.

T: But you're willing to.

P: Oh, without a doubt.

T: Good. So what I want you do is to think of that memory again, and notice what's happening in your body.

P: I definitely notice the anxiety there.

T: Then we're ahead of the game, then. But do you take ownership of the fact that you didn't address it in a constructive way?

P: I can't remember.

T: Did I say you should ignore your anxiety? Did I say you should "keep on truckin'"?

P: No.

T: What did I say you should be?

P: Be aware of it.

T: And be kind.

P: Yes, you did.

T: See, that's hard to remember, isn't it?

P: Yeah.

T: Because that's not the way you been doing it, right?

P: Nope.

T: That's what you're sad about . . . that you've treated yourself with neglect and a kind of meanness—putting yourself down whenever your emotional part gets stirred up.

P: Well, it was probably in looking to give you the right answer.

T: Putting pressure on yourself again. Because what is the "right" answer? The right answer is what you feel. That's the only right answer. See how that's going to lead you away from the truth of your own feeling? If you make it about you and me, and you trying to give me the right answer—already you're starting to treat me like I was your father and you're afraid of me. Do you see that?

P: Mmhm. Well, I guess the right answer was, in trying to get in touch with those feelings from that moment, I'm getting very anxious.

T: Having a spike of anxiety. It's a really quick spike of anxiety in you.

Mental confusion and physical agitation—keep that in your mind, OK?

P: Keep in my mind . . . ?

T: The two places it goes. The mental and the physical.

P: The mental, I really pick up on—the confusion and stuff. The physical, I was aware of that.

T: That's perfect. Now, take yourself back to that memory again, and is that memory a happy memory that you're sharing with me?

P: No.

T: What was it about that memory that you didn't really like? The part of the experience that you . . .

P: Well, I'm feeling that anxiety come in.

The therapist has worked in the triangle of conflict and drew the patient's attention to the causality of his anger, anxiety and mental confusion.

T: That's great. And your job is?

P: To be aware of it.

T: And?

P: To not be mean to myself.

T: Which is called being kind. It's safe to feel your feelings here. I don't think it was safe your whole life to feel your feelings.

P: No.

T: So you see the problem?

P: Mmhm. I understand it.

T: Good. What's that like for you?

P: Understanding the problem? Well, you know, I do feel a little enlightened. Maybe like there's a little light at the end of the tunnel.

T: So hope is what you're experiencing?

P: Yes.

The patient has assimilated the understanding that he cowers with fear at the prospect of facing his true feelings in front of his projected "father."

Vignette 7

Overcoming Defenses Against Anxiety: We are one hour and two minutes into the session.

T: And I just want to ask you again, when the sad feeling is here for you, how is that for you? How does that feel for you?

P: It's fine.

T: It's a relief, is it?

P: (Cries.) Yeah, it's fine. I'm fine with it. I feel like I'm getting stuff out. It feels like it maybe takes some pressure away.

T: Is the confusion gone for you?

P: Yeah, it calms me down.

T: And the muscles feel more relaxed?

P: Yeah.

T: So if we just say it over and over again, you being in touch with your true feelings defeats the anxiety, defeats the confusion, defeats the tension, and makes all of those other compensations—the putting pressure to perform, being detached from your emotions, being compulsive about achieving—it makes all of those things elective. You don't have to do any of those. You can do them if it suits you, but you don't *have* to do them. Do you see the difference?

P: Mmhm.

The patient's punitive superego is identified and temporarily made ego-dystonic, which allows him to be kind to himself and allows the unconscious therapeutic alliance to emerge. He feels grief for the abuse he suffered as a child and for the suffering his punitive part promotes.

Vignette 8

Grief about Self-Destructive Defenses: After a fifteen-minute break, the patient talks about his failed marriage and the lack of intimacy he has felt in other relationships. We are ninety minutes into the session.

T: Now I'm seeing a sad feeling coming up.

P: Yeah, I don't know what to . . .

T: Try not to judge it. Just feel it.

P: And it was just a feeling again of being alone. And it's funny, y'know, when I talked to you on the phone, you asked me a question about whether I wanted to be a Playboy—going from girl to girl, and I said no, I want a relationship. I want a meaningful relationship with someone, and I started thinking about that. And since I talked to you on the phone, I've been thinking about that. It's exciting, y'know, meeting someone new and all that stuff, but just in talking here today, it's become clear, I probably need it more than most—a meaningful, close relationship.

T: OK, that's all true, but what about the sad feeling? Let's give that some airtime, too. What was making you sad?

P: Just being alone.

T: I thought part of it was that, at this moment, we had a mutual understanding of the problem. Remember, when you were leading me, you were talking about the rationalization, and you got it—the light bulb clicked in your mind.

P: (Cries.) I don't know, maybe I just got it. Just thinking that I've been hurting myself. I'm not sure.

T: That's OK. Just let the sad feeling of the man who's been hurting himself, let that sink in. I don't think there are any maybes about the fact that you've been sabotaging your happiness. This has been a long-term problem for you.

P: (Pause.) Yeah, I think I've put everyone's feelings ahead of my own, but then sometimes I think of myself as so self-centered. Y'know, it's so confusing.

T: But right now we're thinking about the self-destructive part of you that deprives you of the thing in your life that you more than anything else. And how mean and cruel that that is of you, towards you?

Vignette 9

De-repression of the Core Neurotic Forces: The patient remembers driving with his family as a child. He sees his father beating his mother, while he and his brother sit terrified in the back seat. He expresses regret that he didn't tell his father to stop. We are now ready for a direct view of the pathogenic forces of his unconscious. We explore his repressed murderous impulses toward his father. We are three hours into the session.

T: What did you really want to do to your father?

P: Maybe I did tell him to stop.

T: But would that have worked?

P: No.

T: What would you have had to have done to make your mother and your brother safe?

P: Kill him.

T: So picture that. How would you have had to kill him?

P: Get the car off to the side of the road.

T: And then do what?

P: (Pauses.) Shoot him.

T: With what?

P: A gun. Pistol.

T: What size? Small? Big?

P: Small. Medium.

T: Where?

P: In the chest?

T: Show me where on you.

P: (Hits chest.)

T: Right where the pain is, right.

P: (Nods.) In the heart.

T: And what's that feel like, when you see the bullet go in his heart?

P: Sad. (Cries profusely.)

T: Let yourself feel the sadness.

P: It feels sad. Y'know, I was sad when he died. I felt sorry for him.

T: Well, the sadness is not just for him; it's for you.

P: Him and me.

T: Yeah, because how many children want to feel like murdering their father? Not many, right?

P: (Cries deeply.) It's the only way I could've stopped him.

T: And the guilt over wanting to murder him is the guilt that causes you to sabotage your life, to not give yourself what you've wanted in your life. You're punishing yourself.

P: I never thought of murdering him.

T: You thought of murdering him a thousand times.

The therapist has confronted the patient with his defense of denial of his murderous rage against his father as revealed by his own words: "Kill him. It's the only way I could've stopped him." The sobbing begins with deep heaving breath indicating the passage of unconscious guilt to consciousness. Freud's described obstacle to making guilt conscious has been overcome.

P: (Cries in anguish) There was night after night, we would just be in my bedroom, and we would just hear him beating my mom.
T: So we have to come to a stop today. I know this is very difficult to face all these complex feelings in one big sitting, but I find that it's better to get all the cards out on the table at the beginning, so you have an idea of what you have to face with me for the rest of the week. And you can't deny the murderous part of your feelings toward your father anymore.
P: (Cries)

After a three-hour session of unlocking, the patient and the therapist have undone the introjective identification with the patient's father. They have unmasked the punitive superego as the cruel and sadistic father whom he loved but murdered.

Next is a vignette of working through that begins at hour six on day three of therapy.

Vignette 10

Establishing an Unconscious Working Alliance: The patient begins the session by continuing to explore the impact his father's cruelty had on him. We are six minutes into the session.

P: I got that all the time.
T: OK. What did he say to you?
P: He said, "The best thing going to come for you is a cop's bullet coming into your head. And you'll be lying in a ditch with a cop's bullet in your head. You're useless. You're scum."
T: You call that positive or you call that negative?
P: That's terribly negative.
T: OK, so you see where the negativity inside comes from?
P: Mmhm.

T: Where does it come from?

P: It was drilled into my whole life.

T: By?

P: My dad.

T: So, you see, the problem is, you've internalized his attitude toward you. For you, it's one step forward, and two steps back. You take a step forward, and he's saying to you, "You worthless son of a bitch, you don't deserve this success. This success is like a suit of clothes that doesn't fit you. Take it off." You follow me? You get pounded by him.

P: I go for what naturally should be mine, and as quick as I go to get it . . . y'know, I can relate to it throughout my whole life. With relationships with other people, feeling that no one liked me, and I know it's ridiculous.

T: What you do is you project your internalized attitude, your father's attitude—you take it and project it into the mind of someone who wants to be your friend.

P: . . . I'm projecting in that, I'm thinking that's what you're feeling, but you're not really feeling that.

T: I'm not really feeling that, but that's what you're thinking I'm feeling. Does that fit?

P: That makes sense, yeah.

T: But does that not only make sense, but does it *fit* what really goes on in your life? Because I want you to see how awful that is of you to do that to you. Because all that does is make you isolated from people who really do love you. It makes you pull away.

P: Yeah.

T: Do you see the destructive nature of that particular mechanism?

P: Mmhm. Yeah.

T: When you understand it, and when you evaluate it as an intelligent person like you are, is it kind or cruel to you?

P: It's very cruel . . . makes life impossible to enjoy.

The patient consolidates insight into the way projecting his punitive superego sabotages his closeness with others. He is less and less identified with his superego. We are now twenty minutes into hour six and we explore his mixed feelings towards his father. He recalls his father's cruelty towards his sister (who eventually committed suicide in the family's garage), his younger brother (now an alcoholic) and toward his mother who he observed being beaten and sexually assaulted by his father.

Following an hour (hour seven of therapy), the patient feels his rage beneath his anxiety when exploring his feelings about his father's mistreatment of his loved ones. He visualizes savagely attacking his father and viciously murdering him, then driving him to the desert to die all alone. He fantasizes that he would drive away with no final words. We are one hour into the session, beginning hour seven of treatment.

T: How are you feeling as you get back in the car? Are you just watching him die?

P: No, I just want to get out. Get away. It's ugly. I want to get back to the ocean.

T: I think that's a positive idea.

P: I just want to get back to the ocean. (Cries very deeply with severe access to pain)

T: Is it hard to leave him?

P: No.

T: Good.

P: (Cries) I just think how fucking mean he was to me, to some little kid who loves water, so full of fucking life. I just feel sorry for myself.

T: As you should. As you should.

P: (Cries)

T: Would you tell me about the ocean?

P: I'm at the ocean.

T: Tell me about it.

P: It's alive. It's beautiful. I feel free. (Cries) I'm the ocean man . . . I love the ocean.

T: Things are as they should be. He's at the desert; you're at the ocean, and you love it there. And you're feeling free. So all the negativity is expunged from your mind? There's nothing between you and the ocean anymore?

P: Now I'm walking on the beach. I'm running on the beach.

T: . . . Your goal is to sustain this way of being, this way of feeling—connected to the beach, running on the beach. You're here, the negativity is shriveling up in the desert. I mean, it's just going to be a skeleton pretty soon.

P: It is already. Shriveled skin and bone.

T: And that's feeling how?

P: Freedom. He's gone.

The patient experiences complete freedom from domination of the ego part by his superego part. He replaces his devaluing and sadistic superego with love for himself as a child. He no longer projects that part of him into the therapist.

In hours eight through fourteen the patient has multiple breakthroughs by exploring the triangle of conflict. He encounters pockets of rage towards his mother for her passivity, self-neglect and alcoholic co-participation with his father. He fantasizes murdering her with a vicious attack, and buries her in the backyard of his home with love and tenderness. He also relived the burial of his dead sister, buries her on a cliff overlooking the ocean, and grieves for her pain. He also addressed his guilt over not protecting her. On the night before session four—hour 12 he reported having spontaneous breakthroughs while on a treadmill at his hotel. He felt his rage and saw images of him murdering his mother and father on the wall. He felt pride that he had addressed his rage independently. We see a vignette of his termination session. We enter at forty-five minutes into hour fourteen.

Vignette 11

Termination

T: So, give me an update on where we're at. We're in the home stretch, so . . . ?

P: Yeah. It was an interesting night. I ended up back at my place, and I started doing a bit of writing. Something just hit me like a ton of bricks, and how important it was. I wrote in real big letters like this, how important it is for me *to take care of myself.* And I made a promise—I wrote down, "You are a big, strong, competent, able, smart man with means, no matter what it takes; you care of that little kid." And it gave me such hope. And during this negative time, I was feeling, like last night, for a

> couple hours . . . well, here I am, it's Friday, it's tomorrow, and I'm going to be going back to my home. Y' know, you're in there, and you're seeing yourself, and what happens after that. I don't worry about that now. Because I really, really believe it's lasting now, and I'm starting to answer some of my own questions. And this morning, stuff came into my head—questions—and I'm answering them.

The patient went on to express gratitude and warmth to the therapist about his efforts on the patient's behalf and good-byes were exchanged. Follow-up arrangements were consolidated.

The patient, between sessions, consolidated his commitment to and practice of self-care. His identification with the punitive superego ended. He returned home and three months later reported freedom from his anxiety, depression, life-long negativity and called up his prior girlfriend, re-instituted dating and has set a wedding date.

Introjection, Identification, and Superego Formation

The above transcript describes the process of identifying an ego-syntonic superego in block therapy and rapidly deconstructing it. Doing therapy in this way, after Davanloo, promotes the development of an unconscious therapeutic alliance and accelerates the working-through process. The unconscious therapeutic alliance refers to the dormant force in the patient's instinctual self towards self examination, self care, and curious self exploration without judgment. As therapy progressed the patient became more interested in his own unconscious, less terrified of his destructive impulses and more able to accept and tolerate closeness.

The metapsychology of ISTDP offers a useful framework to apply certain techniques that allow for symptom relief as well as character change. Many therapists have modified Davanloo's original approach and techniques and have met with success in their modifications. However, a common feature of these variations of ISTDP therapy is that patients become aware that they are participating in an unconsciously organized drama, one as compelling as Freud's speculation of the "Ur-Patricide" with which we began this paper, in which a patient's healthy part is the protagonist which, energized by an appropriate motive (*e.g.*, freedom, not vengeance), does battle with a punitive antagonist and conquers it (Adler 2007). As the patient develops insight into his internal drama, he experiences a catharsis of intense feelings—ranging from grief to joy—which engenders a new and vitalized sense of self, and the ability to pursue a future free of self-inflicted pain.

If one Greek myth, the bloody and tragic Oedipus saga, was the beginning of modern psychology's appreciation of the superego's power, another Greek myth, the story of Orestes and the Furies, may be its fitting conclusion. Orestes killed his mother and her lover to revenge their murder of his father. The Furies, that trio of merciless goddesses who relentlessly pursued those who transgressed the law or the moral order, were lured to him by the smell of his mother's blood. They haunted him day and night, whispering a song only he could hear. They were inescapable and deadly. Against such a punitive force, Orestes' end seems certain. Then something remarkable happens. Athena, goddess of wisdom, takes pity on him, and recruits ten Athenians to try him. She appoints Apollo, god of medicine and healing, as his advocate. When he wins his case, the Furies assent to leniency and are thenceforth called the Eumenides, the Merciful Ones.

What strikes us in the resolution of this myth is not that the Furies are vanquished, but rather that the relationship between them and our hero can now occur in an altered context. Why did the ancient Greeks make that inspired choice, and why should it still resonate so profoundly several millennia later? In a comment that bridges what the Greeks intuited and what Freud theorized, Fenichel (1945) observed that "the superego is the heir of the parents not only as a source of threats but also as a source of protection and as a provider of reassuring love. Being on good or bad terms with one's superego becomes as important as being on good or bad terms with one's parents previously was." In just that way, the Orestes myth is as good a metaphor of the therapeutic process as one can find, and, more importantly, it surely indicates that, while psychologically-minded myth, and therapeutic theories change with time, our inherent desire for psychological soundness endures.

Understanding and Overcoming Projective Identification in ISTDP

Part I

WITH EMANUEL PELUSO, MFT

In this article the authors describe the mechanism of projection and projective identification as described by Davanloo and others. An initial interview of an illustrative case is presented wherein the mechanism of projection, projective identification and double projective identification is central to the origin and maintenance of the patient's symptoms. The authors emphasize how the techniques of affective experiencing in ISTDP and Attachment-Based Interventions help the patient free himself from the cycle of projection and projective identification. The authors demonstrate how to prevent it or deal with it as it occurs.

Introduction

Patients with personality disorders present for treatment with inflexible adaptive responses, or rigidity. Because their rigidity is ego-syntonic, it remains outside their awareness, so they are trapped in a pattern of automatic and repetitive responses, often to their own disadvantage. Even when these patients are made aware of their self-sabotaging choices they can still remain incapable of an alternative action.

Borderline personality disorder is a significant subset of personality disorders. Although prevalence in the general population is estimated at less than 2 percent (cited in Stone, 2006), it is claimed by some to be the most commonly treated disorder, and among the most difficult to treat (Dingfelder, 2004). Borderline personality disorders can be differentiated into two tiers: high-functioning pathology and low-functioning pathology (Caligor et al., 2007). This correlates with Davanloo's categories of fragile and borderline patients (figure 1).

Figure 1. Davanloo's Spectrum of Psychoneurosis Correlated with Kernberg's Classification

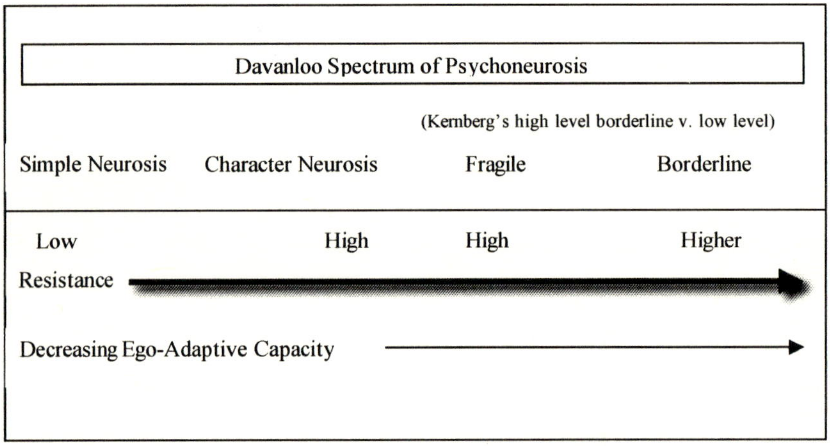

Patients in both tiers display the maladaptive rigidity characteristic of the disorder, but lower functioning patients cannot maintain a consistent sense of self-identity independent of the relationship matrix they are in.

Treating borderline patients presents special challenges. As one writer put it, "They can be quick to open up to a therapist, and perhaps even quicker at shutting down" (Dingfelder, 2004). As the case below illustrates, while they are often hungry for approval, they are also exquisitely sensitive to being rejected or criticized, and their reaction to either can be extreme. Given all this, plus the seeming intractability of their functioning, therapists can easily find themselves in a therapeutic stalemate, or frustrated by insurmountable counter-transference issues. Little wonder, then, that there are only a handful of therapeutic models that attempt to deal with this population—Cognitive Behavior Therapy, Dialectical Behavior Therapy and Psychodynamic Therapies being the most prominent (Stone, 2006).

Patients with borderline personality disorder rely on self/other image distorting defenses: splitting, dissociation and projection, or other "primitive defenses." These defenses support the repression of impulses at extraordinary high cost to the ego: its ability to accurately perceive reality. This is quite different from what we observe in neurotic patients. Borderline patients employ these defenses to avoid any situation that could potentially activate structural conflict.

In order to justify the diagnosis of Borderline Personality Disorder, the therapist must observe the use of splitting (a form of dissociation) and projection as defenses against intra-psychic conflict. This point is crucial. The clinical interview shows these personality disordered patients to have superegos which are punitive in the mistreatment of their emotions and which sustain an inability to perceive others accurately (see figure 2 under "Discussion"). The key diagnostic point in ISTDP is whether the patient responds well (feels and functions better) to the interventions designed to bring the repressed conflictual feelings to the surface. If he does, he is deemed a potentially good candidate for ISTDP, with significant modifications of technique, as the case below demonstrates.

To date, there is no evidence that this approach is superior to other approaches by shortened therapy time or better results—Transference Focused Therapy, Dialectical Behavior Therapy or Mentalization Based Treatment (Kernberg, 2004).

Consistent with other patients on the right side of the spectrum of psychoneurosis, the higher-level functioning patient presented here demonstrates a highly punitive and sadistic superego (figure 1). This case illustrates the inherent dilemma in the treatment of these patients: they are identified with their suffering, and their suffering is what consolidates their identity. A successful treatment of these patients necessitates reformulating their self definition. They need to renounce the introjected sense of self which they absorbed from their caretakers' conscious and unconscious mental construct of them. What can emerge, then, is a repaired, coherent and self compassionate self-identity. The case below is especially complicated, because both caregivers treated the patient and his siblings in a cruel and sadistic fashion, so the patient's self-definition was that of an inherently bad child who deserved punishment. His childhood reality was that psychic pain and love were equivalent.

Table 1 offers a list of the defenses seen in the patient during the course of treatment. He was treated in total with 41 hours of psychotherapy.

Table 1. Defenses Seen in Higher Level Borderline Patients

- Splitting/Dissociation
- Primitive idealization
- Devaluation
- Projection
- Grandiosity/Omnipotent control
- Primitive denial
- Instant repression

The Patient

This annotated case transcript shows the use of Davanloo's approach with a higher functioning patient. The patient presented with panic, depression, substance abuse (alcohol), social isolation, social anxiety, and severe obsessions. He used dissociation and projection to keep his conflictual unconscious impulses and feelings away from consciousness. The transcript shows the subtle ways in which dissociation and projection can potentially block therapeutic progress as the patient ignores his non-verbal signals of anxiety and aggression in the relationship with the therapist. This case also reveals "double projective identification" as first described by Davanloo (personal communication, 1995), meaning that the patient has a punitive superego from both parental introjects. In Davanloo's thoughts the unconscious superego is projected onto the other, the loved order is "murdered" and the other is internalized as yet more superego—doing further damage to the self. Since each of these introjects are potentially activated in the context of a love relationship, the patient self-isolates from intimacy with idealization, devaluation or withdrawal. If the patient does achieve intimacy, it comes at a high prize. The patient develops a more punitive superego and creates symptoms in his partner via projective identification. This is why relationships with these patients are so difficult for them and their partners.

Part I of this two-part article deals with the initial interview.

Getting the Stuck Unstuck

The patient is a forty-two-year old equipment salesman who was referred by a former patient. He is single, never married and lives alone. He is the middle of six children, each described as having severe issues. One sister died from a drug overdose. His father was an alcoholic surgeon who had no interest in his children and drank himself into a stupor nearly every night. His mother was a nurse who gave up her career to have children.

The patient was mentally and physically abused by his mother from age five to mid-teens. She delivered severe physical and psychological punishment for even minor infractions. His father supported her in this and delivered further beatings when he came home at night. If the patient cried when beaten, he would be beaten again until he stopped. When the patient was too old to be beaten, his mother would lock him outside at night in the backyard in order to terrorize him into remorse.

As a sixteen-year-old the patient developed unremitting OCD and was hospitalized in an adolescent psychiatric facility for three months. He never disclosed the abuse. The patient was stuck in his current therapy and suffered from recurrent depression, alcohol abuse, severe social anxiety and hypercritical self-devaluing intrusive thoughts. He is aware that he has an avoidant personality and pleases others no matter what. He had taken antidepressants with only partial relief.

The first vignette is the initial interview in which the therapist asks about the areas of disturbance.

P: The first two off the bat would be . . . I live a life of fear and anger, my most manifested emotions. So that's really it. When I say fear . . . I think it goes back to abandonment issues, so I want your approval, the person's at the gas station approval . . . I want the person that works for me, the person I work for . . . Everyone I meet, at all costs.

T: That's a defense mechanism. You know what I mean?

P: So I don't get hurt first?

T: Right. It gives you control over the interaction.

The ego-syntonic tactical defenses are highlighted and lightly made dystonic.

P: That's true. But it's desperateness. It doesn't feel like control. You know what I mean. It's probably my way of controlling it, but it's desperation in that . . . I'm in sales, and I talk rapidly fast, like someone who's in trouble or about to get hit.

T: It's called galloping, consistent with a state of anxiety, you have rapid speech. So you have a very strong anxiety, stimulated by interpersonal interactions. Very rapid spike, very long duration, doesn't come down to baseline very easily. And you suffered with this, for how long?

P: I would guess, since I was a little kid. That's how our household was. It was extremely abusive, physically and verbally, primarily from the mom, where anything could go wrong in a second.

T: While you're telling me this, what age are you thinking of yourself as in your mind?

P: As far back as I can remember, so I would say I feel like a frozen four-year-old child. I don't know where that number came from.

The second ego-syntonic defense of rapid speech is identified.

T: Problem number two was anger. So could you tell me about problem number two?

P: It's what I call "chicken-poop" anger. The term would be passive-aggressive, meaning it's not face to face. But I will chew someone out in my car who's driving to slow. Whatever. I think if someone cut me off, I'll be just screaming so bad that my throat ends up hurting. To where I'll almost explode, literally. If someone tells me, "No" . . . And it's an anger that someone has to pay. It's an attacking anger. It might be verbally, where I try and demean somebody. And it's never been physical, but in my mind I'll play it out as physical, all the way to killing that person. Playing through a scenario . . .

T: So it's kind of like a revenge, retaliation . . . that they're paying in some fashion or other . . . for having made you feel bad.

P: Bad. Exactly. But it is definitely intentional and definitely attacking.

The third defense of displacement is addressed. His use of the term "chicken poop" reflects an ego-dystonic defense. We continue ten minutes into the session.

T: And how about in your personal relationships, as far as intimacy and closeness with someone?

P: What's happened is, the relationship starts, I couldn't keep my hands off them . . . and just crazy about them and vice versa, and a lot of fun and then . . . twice this has happened . . . with girls that have actually stuck around for six month . . . I've never been in a relationship . . . over a year, but this has happened twice . . . where I didn't want them touching me. Same beautiful girl I was with seven months ago, I didn't want them touching me. I didn't want anything physical to do with them, I no longer found them desirable, and just was looking for another girl. Even though this one I put on a pedestal. So, there has been no intimacy.

T: So you go from idealization about their beauty and they make you look good, in other people's eyes and all of that stuff, to devaluation, where you push them away and make them feel as though they're not desirable any longer.

P: Yeah, I think it's some sort of defense mechanism. Maybe I hurt them before they hurt me.

The fourth defense of idealization/devaluation/distancing from real relationships is labeled.

T: OK, those are the three areas we've talked about: anxiety, anger, relationships. Any other problems we need to address. Drugs? Alcohol?

P: Yes, alcohol. I would guess you could say I'm a functioning alcoholic. I keep it to the weekend, for the most parts. When I drink, I drink to be somewhere else.

T: To escape.

P: It's not to enjoy the taste of alcohol; it's to be somewhere else. To be drunk. To escape. I get a little courage when I'm drinking . . .

T: The anxiety lowers.

P: Yes, exactly. But most of time it leaves me really depressed. Because it's a depressant. Surprise, surprise.

The fifth defense is use of alcohol to escape, a result of projective identification with his father.

The patient says that anytime he is alone, even sitting in the waiting room for this session, he experiences deep sadness.

P: To me it just feels like a caving in. It'll happen anywhere, especially at my desk, where I'll just put my head in my hands and just slowly go into almost comatose state where I just can't go on. It's deep sadness. It's a combination of despair, sadness. Not much fear. It's just a . . . sadness is the word that keeps coming up.
T: So a sad feeling starts to . . .
P: A hopeless feeling. You're sad about something.
T: Are you in touch with it as we're talking?
P: If I think about it, sure. I can go there pretty quick, just because it's so frequent.

The patient uses the sixth and seventh defense of instant repression and depression to avoid his grief. He completes the diagnostic phase confirming low ego-adaptive capacity. The trial therapy begins.

T: It seems to me we have a couple of things going on at the same time. I mean, that's normal. OK? One is, when you're just with yourself, your feelings start to push themselves toward the surface. Now is the process of feeling your own emotions a trigger for anxiety in you?
P: I would think so.
T: OK, so take a very careful inventory of the symptoms you're having of anxiety right now. What are the symptoms of anxiety, that you're having?
P: I guess I'm retracting. I'm leaning back in the chair and just real intimidated . . . so I'm kind of gripping—not saying that I shouldn't be—but that's what I'm doing.

"Intimidated" reflects that projection is perhaps occurring—it is a key to explore the transference.

T: Good, you're doing what I'm asking you to do. You're giving me an inventory of your symptoms.

P: It's very tight and defensive, like, don't get any closer. Not that we're going to fight. But just, I'm not comfortable.

"Not that we're going to fight" is classical negation and reflects the denial mechanism around his aggression which is mobilized in the transference.

T: Yeah. I agree with what you're saying. The issue is about emotional closeness. Emotional closeness brings up more and more feeling in you. And the more emotion that comes up, creates more and more anxiety in you. It's a cycle. It's a circle. So you have to push either escape on your end, to retreat, or push me away. One or the other.
P: Yes.
T: Otherwise the pain becomes intolerable. Is that correct?
P: Yes, I can't stay in . . .
T: So you have a lot of what I call motor tension in your body, right now.
P: Yeah, I do.
T: Do an inventory. Where does it start?
P: In the jaw, and the upper back. I frequently have issues with a pinched nerve in my back.
T: But you started to notice it first in the jaw? Do you ever notice it hands, arm, shoulders? Does it ever start in hands, arms, shoulders?
P: It seems more up here. That and my stomach.
T: The stomach? That is somatic anxiety.
P: I'll tighten it almost like you're going to hit it, but you're not.
T: So you're having tension in your stomach wall.
P: Almost like I'm intentionally tightening it like a defense. Like I'm going to get hit. To protect myself.

This is more evidence of denial, projection and projective identification.

T: Anything else?
P: What I also get when I stop and be with myself . . . Especially if I do it in a safe environment, me in my room, following a meditation tape . . . and with my therapist, because we were doing some inner stuff, first thing, and this has been seven sessions in a row, what happens is, the stomach again, an energy of wanting to cry comes up and is always suppressed. I'll put my tongue on top of my mouth. I'll shut it down in the

jaw, I'll focus on it and it'll go away and within thirty seconds, just a whimpering, a cry wants to come out.

T: You really have good somatic awareness of your physical state changes, and you're noticing a relationship between a sad feeling, and the use of anxiety and tension as a way of crippling your ability to experience the sad feelings. It stops at all costs. So you're starting to really see those relationships.

P: Yeah, just because I've been practicing them. At other times, if I sit, and I can get through a couple of minutes, which is difficult, I'll start like this (he hand trembles).

T: Trembling.

P: It's almost like a release of energy, but I'm guessing. I'll tighten up. It can go on, if I let it.

T: I discourage you from thinking of it as anything but a release of anxiety. You're releasing anxiety through the trembling. I don't consider anxiety to be a constructive energy. I consider anxiety to be an energy, but it's a destructive energy. Do you see what I'm saying? You're discharging anxiety by that motion. Some people do it like this (shakes foot).

P: It's funny . . . it'll come out. There's not something I'm not cognizant . . .

T: It's a discharge.

P: Is that what it is? Sometimes it'll be a leg. If I let it go and focus on being calm and breathing, it kind of takes on a life of its own. I've always wondered what it is.

T: It's a discharge. Of anxiety. You have what I would describe as crippling levels of anxiety.

P: Yes, I would agree. Crippling is a great way to put it.

T: And you're looking and acting like a cripple who's incapacitated.

P: It goes like that. If I played through it . . .

T: So that's really important to understand. And the second part of it is, just like alcohol, anxiety is a way of escaping. Anxiety is way of suppressing emotions. Because you're saying to me, in very astute terms, your therapist has helped you, by encouraging you to experience more feelings. Anxiety is a way to suppress feelings. The irony is, you're between a rock and a hard place. If the therapy is encouraging you to feel more, but there's another, less healthy part, that is discouraging you from feeling your emotion, you don't have any place to go. You see you're trapped?

P: Yeah, that's exactly it. And that's why I have a shelf full of self-help books with book-markers in them. Because I have the energy . . . I want to get better . . .

T: The healthiest part of you wants to feel your feelings and overcome your difficulties.

P: Exactly, but then something sabotages it every time.

T: Every single time.

P: Every single time. Whether I loose interest right away . . . And that part is stronger, I believe.

T: What do you mean? The sabotage is stronger?

P: Yes.

T: Well in a sense it is, and in a sense it's not. The way it is, is that you haven't been able to overcome it. Bu the healthy part of you is determined to overcome it or you wouldn't be seeking my assistance. The reason you're here is because you're sick and tired of the unhealthy part of you dominating the part of you that wants to heal.

P: Yes, that's 100% of it.

T: Yeah. There's that struggle there. As long as you and I are allied on the basis of the healthy part of you, we can defeat this crippling side of you, the side that wants to escape from facing your true feelings.

P: Yes.

We continue forty minutes into the session.

T: So which side do you wish to ally yourself with?

P: That's a good question? The obvious answer would be the good side. But there's also part of me that wants to hold on to it.

T: But what would happen if you give in to that side?

P: To the good side?

T: To the side that wants to hold on.

P: It would be the same non-existent, fear-filled lifestyle.

T: OK, but more microscopically. What would happen in our interactions? How would you feel when you leave here?

P: Frustrated.

T: Defeated.

P: Exactly. Like that was my last shot.

T: One more person who's . . .

P: That's exactly it . . . it didn't work. There's no help for me.

T: And is that the outcome you want?
P: No, by no means.

The therapist uses a mild "head-on collision with the patient's alliance with his punitive superego and cements the therapeutic alliance by allying with the patient's desire to face his feelings.

T: Because if we have a healthy alliance here, you and me . . . we're going to ally together to do what?
P: To diminish the bad side.
T: And, to encourage you to feel your emotions. So what are your emotions right at this minute?
P: My emotions are . . . that's a thought . . . I can't believe this.
T: What are your emotions?
P: That I'm stuck.
T: You wouldn't be in this chair if you weren't stuck. That's no big revelation.
P: Yeah, it's true.
T: I asked you what are your emotions?
P: My emotions are . . . An anger. An anger toward the bad side again. It might even be at my good side, for being so weak. I guess more at being such a wimp. For being a lot worse than I say. For being such a fuckin' pussy. Such a friggin' weak little piece of crap. That's where I'm going at it, right now.
T: You're saying, for taking a castrated position.
P: Yes, and pissed off at my good side for being so damned weak. And getting bullied, and getting its ass kicked, over and over. And here's a chance to do something . . .

Although the therapist was unaware (consciously) of the target of his rage, it becomes clear that the rage is at his passive father who was bullied by his mother.

T: But I have to tell you something. Your anger is part of your healthy side. Isn't it?
P: Because I can use it . . .
T: Because your anger is part of your healthy side. It's one of your feelings. So describe it. How does it feel? How do you experience your anger inside?

P: I want to attack it. I want something to pay. I've been gritting my teeth. Right now I'm holding back.

T: So you're telling me you have actually a rage inside.

P: Yes, exactly. If I could elbow this . . . I want something to break. I wouldn't want to hit a punching bag. I'd want to throw that . . .

T: You have a destructive impulse inside.

P: I want something to pay, whether it's the phone . . . Doing twenty push-ups won't get it out. I want to attack something right now.

T: So could we take a look at that? I'd like you to picture, in your mind's eye, like we did before . . . the attack that you'd like to make. Image it in your mind. What do you see yourself doing, to express this impulse? It's full destructive power?

P: It would be to elbow that, because I think it's glass. There'd be noise. Throw this lamp against the wall, just start throwing things. Smashing and noise. Things are breaking.

T: I understand. But you also said, you want someone to pay. Remember when you had the rage? It's always a retaliatory rage, isn't it?

P: Yes, always an attack, retaliatory . . .

T: So picture, against whom you'd like to direct this.

P: It's blocking. There's nothing yet.

T: I understand. Take all the time you need. Just whoever comes into your thoughts.

P: Inside I'm cursing at someone, but I'm not sure who it is yet. Calling them motherfuckers.

T: Did you have a spike of anxiety there for a second?

P: Yeah. Something's trying to quench my anger, something saying "Don't get angry."

T: Crippling you. Why do you have to cripple your anger? What would happen if you don't?

P: I don't know if I could stop it.

T: What would be the worst thing you could do if you didn't stop your anger with the anxiety? If you didn't obey the destructive side of you?

P: Maybe I'd hurt myself.

T: Stop with hurt yourself! What would be the worst thing you could do to someone else?

P: The anxiety's up again, saying, "Calm down, don't . . ."

T: Saying, "Don't answer the guy's question?"

P: Almost like it's making me really tired. I shut down.

T: That's terrific. Not that that's happening. But your powers of observation are enormously strong.

P: Good.

T: They really are. That's actually the mechanism of depression that you're interrupting. Shutting down your aggression is the way people create mental depression.

P: Oh really. I have depression up the wazoo.

T: You're showing me. And do you remember what the specific challenge was I was putting on the table? You have a rage inside of you, right? You felt it.

P: Yes.

T: I saw it come up, from here. It went up, out your arms. You were wanting to hit, smash, hurt, destroy. Correct? And what did I ask you?

P: To play them through.

T: Toward?

P: Someone.

T: And who do you have all this rage against?

Each of his defenses begins to interfere with the continuity of his emotional experiencing. Despite his excellent ability to experience the impulse it is dissociated from the object (splitting). He keeps himself ignorant of the object of the impulse. Please note that all this work could have unfolded in the transference with the therapist as the target of the aggression, but this is really unnecessary as he is making the implicit T-P links as he feels the impulse.

P: I know it's my mom, my dad. Especially my mom. But I'm not visualizing attacking her . . .

T: Let's start with your dad.

The therapist's unconscious had picked up the link between rage at his passivity and the projective identification with his father.

P: Him, would be the fucking wimp that I just detested and was talking about. And probably inherited from him.

T: Or identified with.

P: Identified with. He had two moods: silence or rage. Only time he made contact was when my mom said we were bad, then he had to hit us because she said so. Then he just went about his business after that.

T: How do you see, in your mind's eye, your attack against him?

P: I would do . . . right now I would shove him against the wall. I'd head butt him, so I'd smash his nose. Then I'd start throwing elbows, just coming right back, until he was nothing. If he dropped, I'd pick him up again, I'd head-butt him again, knee him in the groin, in the stomach, break his ribs. I wouldn't stop.

T: The more precise and specific you can be, the better. I can see a spike of anxiety. Let's not ignore it, but use the power of your intelligence and understanding of how important it is for us to examine your aggression, and understand the details of your aggression. Not any cover-up or superficial . . . but a very detailed . . . I see this as being, in my mind, as a very powerful attack: head-butt, crushing his ribs, and every time he tries to become passive you pick him up and give him another dose of . . .

P: Yeah, like you're not going to get out of this easy. I'm not done with you, even though you're knocked out, I'm going to pick you up and see how you like it. See how you like being defenseless and whipped and screamed at. Call him a piece of crap. You're not going to get away with it. So don't try to pass out or drop. You're going to stay there and take it. Like I stood there and took it from you.

T: You're experiencing toward your father kind of a torturous rage that has a huge power, a desire to crush and hurt him, inflict pain, and not allowing him to escape into passivity.

P: Yes.

T: And what does he look like in this assault that you're imagining?

P: Terrified. Weak. Defenseless. All the opposite of what he was to me when he was beating the crap out of me.

T: I hear all that and it's fine. But describe the extent of his physical injuries that you've inflicted on him. If your anxiety spikes, it's fine. Let me know. If your head gets fuzzy or any kind of . . . because it's not my intention to ignore your anxiety. I want us to really lower it through our commitment. Because I sense there's more brutality in you. I sense you're holding back. So if you don't hold the beast back, if you don't cripple the beast inside of you with anxiety . . . Because you said: "If I let him out of the cage . . ." So let's look at that. What do you see the beast inside of you doing? This angry, raging . . .

P: I'm torn between visualizing myself as a kid, getting up off the bed when I've been whipped, or right now doing it to the 72-year-old man he is.

T: It doesn't make any difference. Just stay with the task at hand. So, this man is here in the chair, and the picture that would give you the most satisfaction.

P: If he were here in that chair, I would lunge. I'd go right for the throat. I'd push the chair over, and just start throwing overhand rights. Repeatedly, repeatedly. And I could see him trying to stop it. And I'd tell him . . .

T: But you said lunge for the throat. When you say that, what are you describing? What impulse? Feel that full, very basic animal urge. Without crippling yourself. What do those hands want to do?

P: That's the quickest point I can do pain, as opposed to going to his eyes. I'd put my knuckles right to his throat.

T: Yeah, that's what I was sensing. So feel the power of that. Right there, what's that feel like? Hands on his throat, what would those thumbs do?

P: Press in. Fucking go in. I'd like to pop his neck.

T: What's that feel like, when you feel his neck pop?

P: Then I'd get mad. It would be like, you motherfucker.

T: Yeah, there'd be a release. "You motherfucker."

P: Then I'd go to . . . Oh, God! (He clenches his fist very tightly and bends forward.)

T: You'd just what? You'd just what?

P: I'd scream so loud!

T: Yeah, but what would you do to his throat? With those powerful arms. Look at the power of them. Your forearms, fists. Look at the strength you have.

P: I just . . .

T: You just what?

P: I'd rip his throat open. I'd dig into it and rip it open.

T: Let yourself feel the full extent . . .

P: I'd spit on him. Out of disgust. Just fucking disgust. Looking down at him . . .

T: He dies how? With pain?

P: I think I'm not done with him yet. I just take his jaw and snap it, snap his neck. And then he'd be dead.

T: And what does that feel like?

P: It feels like I'm not done. I'd want to get up and just jump on top of his stomach, just grind him, grind him. Just fucking grind him!

T: Crush his stomach . . .

P: Crush his stomach, his ribs and organs, till he's no more. Till he's just mush. Then I'd go to his rib cage and I'd jump in with two feet up and down, just stamp on him. Then I'd pull aside and take his head and I'd kick it so it snaps again, spit on him again. Now I'm just full of disgust, toward him. A feeling of . . .

T: Describe his corpse, how it looks.

P: I can see his stubbled, bearded face.

T: And the feeling that you get?

P: The feeling is, I'm not sure of the words, but why did it have to end like this? It didn't have to be this way. It could have been so much better. I'm not sure if that' passivity or . . .

T: No, no. That's your healthy part. That's a sad and painful feeling of regret. Tell him how you wanted . . .

P: You missed out on the relationship of a lifetime (with tears). You died an empty soul, a frightened little kid. You could have had me your whole life.

T: So you grieve for not having had a close, intimate relationship with your father. You're left with the grief.

P: Yeah, now it's just the sadness. I'm looking down, knowing he's gone. You're just a lost soul. I wish I could have helped you with your pain.

T: So you have mixed feelings toward your father. On one hand you want to brutally murder your father and torture and crush him and make him feel total subjugation to your rage.

P: Yes.

T: On the other hand, you feel a deep, deep longing for what could have been.

P: And the disgust . . . No, no . . . the sadness of what he wasted. What I could have offered to him. What I tried to, so desperately, over and over. Now he's just a dead corpse.

T: I would like you to notice how low your anxiety is.

P: Yeah, it is. Very calm, actually.

T: How do you feel about that?

P: I love this feeling. It feels like I'm my age. Meaning . . . I'm forty-two.

I'm a man. It feels like I'm a man. It just feels like . . . it feels like there's no anxiety. I talk slower. There's no reason to impress, no reason to . . . worry and fear. That's how it is. Just a nice calmness. It's really nice.

The patient has a positive reaction to the unlocking indicating that he is a candidate for this approach. We continue one hour and twenty minutes into the session.

T: But look at the corpse. Describe him from head to toe. What he looks like.
P: His head's to the side, eyes are closed. Mouth's closed, which is weird. His neck is all open, boney, the skeleton.
T: What's he look like?
P: Peaceful, which is really . . .
T: Yeah, but what's he look like? You said you ripped open his throat . . .
P: You can see the corpse, the blood all along the side. He looks like a rag doll. He has no more form in his body. He looks like he's sleeping. It's weird. It doesn't look like he's . . .
T: What's the feeling, when you see your father like that?
P: I'm done with you, is what comes up.
T: That's your thought. I wish that were true, but I don't think that's entirely the truth. What 's the feeling? What does he look like? To me, he looks like a man, when I look at that picture . . .
P: Yeah, he's an adult, sure.
T: He looks like a man who's been attacked by a beast.
P: Yes, mauled. Exactly. His neck looks mauled, and his whole body looks like it was run over by a truck. There's no more form. But his face is fine.
T: And this is a man whom you loved. That's what I'm asking you.
P: Yeah, I . . .
T: So tell me what kind of treatment, a son who mauls his father like an animal from the wild, what kind of life do you think that son deserves?
P: Nothing's coming yet.
T: But you heard the question.
P: Yeah.
T: Repeat it.
P: How I interpret it is, what kind of punishment does a child who just murdered his dad deserve? In brutal and intentional way.

T: What kind of punishment does he deserve? You have a very precise mind. I can't say it any more accurately. Let yourself feel, no matter how painful it is. What comes up? Does he deserve a happy life, a fulfilled life, a life full of love? Women who care about him, and professional success?

P: The feeling that comes up doesn't make sense. He deserves to be set free. That's what the feeling is, he deserves . . .

T: I would agree with you.

P: In other words, the world would understand what a horrible person that dad was. And he deserves . . . I don't feel punishment in this yet.

T: Wait, wait, wait. You're missing the point. There has been thirty-six plus years of punishment. Yes, you do deserve to be set free. You've done your time.

The patient does not experience guilt over the murder. This is an indication of further splitting of the loving part from the hating part and his use of projective identification which will lead to continuing to live a life of suffering.

This ends the first clinical part of a two-part article on undoing projective identification.

Discussion

The focus of this article is undoing projection and projective identification. Both projection and projective identification are seen as defenses to avoid the occurrence of intra-psychic conflict. Classically, projective identification (Ogden, 1982) is the process of splitting off aspects of one's internal experience and projecting them onto another person, so that the projected aspects of the self are experienced as part of the other person. The projecting person acts defensively to shape the other person's reactions nut moreover projective identification creates an altered mental state in the receiver of the projection (Goudsmit, 2008). The receiver's reaction to this is varied, including symptoms, defenses, or even perhaps insight.

So in a sense projection is used to support repression, and thus projection and the cycle of projective identification must be interrupted for ego growth to occur. Because these patients have never developed the capacity to tolerate conflicting emotions, love, hate, sexual desire, guilt, etc—

splitting, dissociation, projection and projective identification are used to protect the ego from having to experience anxiety over the emergence of conflicting emotions into awareness. By definition these patients have limited observing and/or attentive ego functions (ten Have-de Labije, 2001) to regulate anxiety, thus reliance on these anxiety limiting defenses to protect the ego comes at a very high price (Figure 2).

This figure demonstrates the ego-superego-reality relationships of a person with a highly functioning borderline personality organization. Inspection of the diagram shows predominance of splitting, idealization, and projection in order to support repression. This system is very stable over time and highly maladaptive to building close, intimate and satisfying relationships. The diagram shows the way projection and idealization impair the ego's ability to perceive reality in any way that is close to accurate. If we are on the idealized side of the split relationships (left side of diagram) things are perceived as very satisfying. If we are on the punitive side (right side of diagram) things are more hostile and dangerous than

Figure 2. The Way Primitive Defenses Support Repression and Alter Perception of Self and Other—Relationship between Splitting, Projection, Idealization, and Object-Relationship Perception

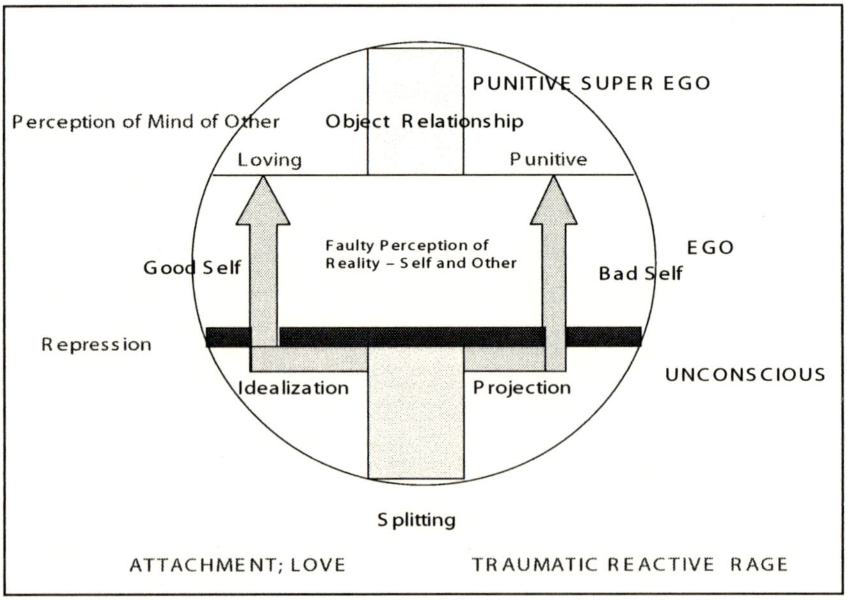

they actually are. These oscillations between polarities are not a function of reality but a function of emotional closeness and/or distance in a relationship; hence they impair ego-adaptive capacity. Furthermore, the superego is just as capricious. It's either very harsh or unconditionally loving to the extreme. The superego itself is projected into the intimate other and the patient responds to its projected superego part. So, if the patient is on the idealizing side, they are very exciting to be with and co-create love, intimacy and sexuality with their "loved one." But, if they are on the punitive side the superego is hostile beyond all bounds and the patient mounts an attack against the "loved one" or hides under a myriad of regressive defenses. This is what makes relationships with these patients so challenging and tumultuous.

Numerous approaches have evolved to the treatment of patients with severe personality disorders. (Leichsenring, 2003, Winston, 1994, Abbass, 2002, Bateman, 2004). The patient in this article qualifies for the higher level "personality pathology" described by Kernberg (2007). This is a difficult-to-treat group of patients and they are challenging to all therapists. The treatment approach of ISTDP has shown utility in this population. ISTDP differs from the other approaches because of its use of systematic clarification of ego defenses to promote affective experiencing in the here-and-now of the therapy.

It is abundantly clear that patients with borderline conditions suffer from low ego-adaptive capacity as well as punitive superegos (see also Figure 1). However, the mechanisms of splitting and projection make the discovery of the punitive part challenging to therapists. Their punitive superegos are difficult to recognize because they are frequently projected into the other. This projection is "seamless" and there is no visible indication that this has occurred. Traditional analytic therapies wait for the evidence that this has occurred to emerge in the form of counter-transference (Bion, 1962a, 1962b).

In this article, we have highlighted the clinical clues that projection has occurred and, had the therapist been inactive, would have eventually led to projective identification and all of its negative results.

Borderline patients have no tolerance of guilt and use punishment of the self as a defense against the experience of complex feelings. Thus, they are prone to all or none thinking and define "self" in the simplistic good or bad axis. The reason for this is the utter lack of compassion that these patients have for their aggressive feelings. This lack of compassion is the internalization of what they perceived of their parent's lack of empathy and compassion for their own destructive feelings. Treatment requires extreme patience to increase ego-adaptive capacity.

On reviewing the above case, it is clear that the patient used the following defenses against feeling: passivity, pleasing, distancing, avoidance, galloping, ignoring, displacement, suppression, escapism (alcohol), depression, idealization, devaluation, dissociation, splitting, projection and projective identification. The evidence for projection is summarized in Table 2.

Table 2. Clues to Projection in the Narrative

- "I guess I'm retracting. I'm leaning back in the chair and just real intimidated . . . so I'm kind of gripping—not saying that I shouldn't be—but that's what I'm doing."
- "It's very tight and defensive, like, don't get any closer. Not that we're going to fight. But just, I'm not comfortable."
- "Almost like I'm intentionally tightening it like a defense. Like I'm going to get hit. To protect myself."

The costs of allowing the projection to continue to the patient are enormous to him and counter any hope for a reconstructive therapy. In his view the world is an unbelievably hostile and threatening environment. All of his difficulties get externalized and he never deals with his inner world which is in continued turmoil. He lives his life, passively and submissively, avoids any conflict with others and he must maintain distance from real relationships—hence idealized relationships or devalued relationships result. His only outlet for his unconscious aggression is temper tantrums in cars and angry retaliatory fantasies towards people who have slighted him. Patients in the lower level personality disordered population often concretely act out their aggression towards others as a logical mobilization of defensive aggression against a perceived persecutor.

Once the projection is blocked, the patient has the opportunity to investigate and become acquainted with his own destructive impulses and the grief, potential guilt and love that reside in his own unconscious.

(Cornelissen, 2005), The very act of taking this approach creates a corrective emotional experience and allows the ego to be enriched and empowered by the affects that are created by relationships, instead of weakened and traumatized by relationships.

Treatment is designed along the lines recommended by ten Have-de Labije's (2001) modification of Davanloo's central dynamic sequence where the installation of a constructive superego for the punitive superego is the first priority. Notice that the model used in the above case is not that of a graded approach (Whitemore, 1996, Abbass, 2007). The patient undergoes a full (major) unlocking of the forces underneath the paternal aspect of the punitive superego. This gives the patient an immediate boost in ego-adaptive capacity (decreased projection) and freedom from one aspect of the projective identification cycle.

The major unlocking of the second introjective system is purposely left for the next session once his ego-adaptive capacity shows improvement.

About the Co-author

Emanuel Peluso is a Marriage and Family Therapist in private practice in Del Mar, California. He is co-author of "Women and Drugs" (CompCare, 1989), and has written numerous articles for professional journals. He studied ISTDP with Dr. Neborsky for five years and practices a variation of it called "Guided Emotional Therapy." He can be reached through his website www.emanuelpeluso.com.

BIBLIOGRAPHY

Abbass, A. (2002) Office based research in ISTDP: data from the first 6 years of practice. Ad Hoc Bulletin of Short-Term Dynamic Psychotherapy 6 (2): 4–15.

Abbass, A., Bechand, D. (2007) Bringing Character Changes With Davanloo's Intensive Short-Term Dynamic Psychotherapy Ad Hoc Bulletin of Short-term Dynamic Psychotherapy Vol 11 (2).

Adler, J.M., Wagner, J.W., McAdams, D.P. (2007), Personality and the coherence of psychotherapy narratives, Journal of Research in Personality, in Press.

American Psychiatric Association Diagnostic and Statistical Manual (2000), 4th edition Washington DC.

Bateman, A. and Fonagy, P. (2004) Psychotherapy for Borderline Personality Disorder: mentalization-based treatment.

Beeber, A.R. (1999), The perpetrator of the unconscious in Davanloo's new metapsychology. Part I: Review of classic psychoanalytic concepts, International Journal of Intensive Short-Term Dynamic Psychotherapy, 13:3, 151–157.

Bion, W.R (1962a) Learning from Experience. London: Heinemann.

Bion, W.R. (1962b) A theory of thinking. International Journal of Psycho-Analysis 43, 306–310.

Caligor, E., Kernberg, O., Clarkin, J. (2007) Handbook of Dynamic Psychotherapy for Higher Level Personality Pathology. American Psychiatric Publishing. Washington, DC.

Cornelissen, K. (2005) Understanding and Undoing Projection: the Alien. Ad Hoc Bulletin of Short-Term Dynamic Psychotherapy, Vol 9 (2). 24–50.

Davanloo, H. (1980). Short-Term Dynamic Psychotherapy. New York: Jason Aronson;

Davanloo, H. (1988b). The technique of unlocking of the unconscious. Part I. International Journal of Short-Term Psychotherapy, 3 (2), 99–121.

Davanloo, H. (1988c). The technique of unlocking of the unconscious. Part II. Partial unlocking of the unconscious. International Journal of Short-Term Psychotherapy, 3 (2), 123–159.

Davanloo, H. (1990). Clinical Manifestations of Superego Pathology. Unlocking the Unconscious. Chichester: Wiley.

Davanloo, H. (1990). Unlocking the unconscious: Chichester, England: John Wiley & Sons.

Davanloo, H. (1995). Intensive short-term dynamic psychotherapy: Spectrum of psychoneurotic disorders. Int. J. Short-term Psychother. 3 (4): 121–232.

Davanloo, H. (2005). Intensive Short-Term Dynamic Psychotherapy. In Kaplan and Sadock's Comprehensive Textbook of Psychiatry: (pp. 2628–2652) Lippincott: Williams and Wilkins.

Dingfelder, S.F. (2004) Treatment for the 'Untreatable'. Monitor on Psychology, 35 (3) 46–48.

Fenichel, O. (1945), The Psychoanalytic Theory of Neurosis. New York: W.W. Norton and Co., p. 105. Cited in Beeber, A.R. (1999).

Freud, S. (?). S.E. XIX, p. 50.

Freud, S. (1897), Anf., 238; Standard Edition, I, p. 265.

Freud, S. (1923), The Ego and the Id. Standard Edition, Strachey, J. Ed. Vol. XIX, 50.

Freud, S. (1924), The economic problem of masochism, Standard ed. Strachey, J. ed. Vol. XIX.

Freud, S. (1926), The question of lay analysis. Standard Edition. Strachey, J. ed. Vol 20, pp. 197–250.

Freud, S. (1933), New Introductory Lectures on Psycho-Analysis. S.E. XXII, p. 129.

Freud, S. (1937), Analysis Terminable and Interminable. Standard edition. Strachey, J. Ed. Vol. XXIII, 209–253.

Freud, S. (1940), An Outline of Psycho-analysis. Standard Edition. Strachey, J. Ed. Vol. XXIII, 205.

Goudsmit, A. (2008) Personal communication "Getting the stuck unstuck" Maastricht, Netherlands Sept. 11, 2008.

Jacobson, E. (1964), The Self and the Object World. New York: International University Press. Cited in Beeber, A.R. (1999).

Have-de Labije, J. ten, Tricht, P. van, (2001), Red and Green Lights on Davanloo's Road to the Unconscious: In The Working Alliance in ISTDP; Whose intrapsychic crisis? ten Have-de Labije, J, ed VKDP, Amsterdam.

Leichsenring, F., Leibing, E. (2003) The effectiveness of psychodynamic therapy and cognitive behavioral therapy in the treatment of personality disorders: a meta-analysis. Am J Psychiatry 160: 1223–1232.

Neborsky, R and Solomon, M. (2001), Attachment Bonds and Intimacy. In Short-Term Therapy for Long-Term Change. W.W. Norton and Co.

Ogden T.H. (1982) Projective Identification and Psychotherapeutic Technique. Jason Aaronson (1993).

Stone, M.H. (2006) Management of borderline personality disorder: a review of psychotherapeutic approaches. World Psychiatry, 5 (1), pp 15–20.

Trilling, L. (1971), The Authentic Unconscious. In *Sincerity and Authenticity,* Harvard University Press.

Whitemore, J. (1996) Paving the Royal Road: An Overview of Conceptual and Technical features in the Graded Format of Davanloo's Intensive Short-Term Dynamic Psychotherapy. Int. J. Short-Term Psychotherapy. 11: 21–39.

Widiger, T. A. & Weissman, M. M. (1991) Epidemiology of borderline personality disorder. Hospital and Community Psychiatry, 42, pp. 1015–1021.

Winston A., Laikin M., Pollack J., Samstag L.W., McCullough L., Muran J.C. (1994) Short-term psychotherapy of personality disorders. American Journal of Psychiatry 151 (2):190{4}.

First published in *Ad Hoc Bulletin of Short-Term Dynamic Psychotherapy: Practice and Theory* 2008, 12, 2.
Reprinted with permission of editor and author(s).

Understanding and Overcoming Projective Identification in ISTDP

Part II: The Man with the Ghost in the Basement and in the Nursery

WITH EMANUEL PELUSO, MFT

This is part two of a two-part article on projective identification. The authors discuss the mechanism of projective identification and its role in creating, maintaining and sustaining character pathology.

Introduction

A new patient walks into your consult room. In the course of the session he unfolds a history of being misunderstood, or neglected, or abused. The suffering in his present life is palpable. Because of your natural compassion, you may feel that being kind, supportive and empathic will help this patient overcome his pain. You may feel, too, that your caring is expressive of that part of you that impelled you into a healing profession. And, in fact, your attentiveness and compassion can offer symptomatic relief. But—as counter-intuitive as it may seem—your kindness may ultimately reactivate the patient's unconscious longings for secure attachment whereby his punitive superego structure can be stimulated rather than alleviated. In short, you have been the object of Projective Identification, and your role as caregiver will only satisfy the patient's most superficial needs, and only do temporarily.

In the 1930s, as psychoanalysis struggled with the phenomenon of negative therapeutic reactions, Anna Freud described the defense mechanism of Identification with the Aggressor to explain why patients adopted negative stances towards themselves or others. (Freud, A., 1936)

Later, Melanie Klein (1946) introduced the term Projective Identification (PI) as a psychological process in which a person's false projections about another causes an interaction in which the other's behavior actually manifests the projections. It is generally believed that this process happens outside the conscious awareness of the parties involved.

In the late 1960s and 70s, Habib Davanloo used the term Projective Identification in his own unique therapeutic approach, ISTDP, considering it as one element of the core of symptom formation. Davanloo based his conception of the unconscious on his observation of the feelings and images that emerged from a direct challenge to the patient's resistance. He called the mutually created state of mind "an unconscious therapeutic alliance." Through the lens of this alliance, he observed that neurotic patients were under the influence of a punitive system of mind called "the Punitive Superego." He saw that the origin of this system was the failed or thwarted attachment relationships that occurred in the patient's developmental past.

Davanloo outlined a process by which a child felt rage, and then guilt, over retaliatory-destructive impulses/feeling-images toward the offending parent. He noted that these patients built a self-destructive system of defenses to protect the attachment figure from being harmed or destroyed by that rage. This system then became a fixed, rigid and seemingly permanent mental/emotional organization. Most importantly, Davanloo noted, this system increased its destructive power over the ego until it subsumed the entire ego-adaptive self. The ego then became identified with the superego and renounced all longings for attachment security.

Davanloo's concept of Projective Identification, then, expands on Klein's schema in significant ways. Davanloo theorized that a patient misperceives the current attachment relationship as attacking or offending in the same way as the original aggressor; he feels retaliatory murderous rage and in his fantasy "kills" the other. In reaction to this fantasy murder, he feels intense guilt and is compelled to punish the self by re-internalizing the corpse of the murdered attachment figure as a punitive structure of mind that dictates that the patient suffer for his misdeed. After a critical mass of these "murders," the patient's pleasure-seeking ego is replaced with the punitive superego. The Punitive Superego has as many components as there are harmful attachment relationships. The variance of the system across the dynamic range of adaptive to rigid (*i.e.*, punitive) is determined by how much love versus how much trauma occurred in each attachment relationship.

The Developmental Origin of the Superego

Between six and eighteen months of age, children develop specific, fear-alleviating relationships with their primary caregiver. Klein as well as Davanloo saw this developmental relationship as the matrix for superego development, unlike from Freud's view that the superego was a creation of the psyche after successful resolution of the Oedipal conflict around age six.

The Kleinian view was that the quality of the caregiver relationship is irrelevant to the formation of the superego since the superego was entirely a function of instinctual endowment. Klein emphasized pre-oedipal unconscious fantasy, which has a significant overlap with Davanloo's view, since the unconscious guilt is the result of the fantasy of the destructive urges. The difference as we see it is that aggression is a result of thwarted developmental archetypical imperatives. Safety, empathy, attunement, stimulation, boundaries, and guidance are all instinctually created requirements in each infant and child. (Stevens, 2005)

With the theories and research of Ainsworth (1978) and Bowlby (1988) it has become self-evident that in healthy parent-child pair bonds there is a highly interactive flow of energy and information. It is a reciprocal relationship where bonds of joy, compassion, empathy and excitement are addressed. Signs of the child's distress evoke comforting reactions in the caregiver. The child learns that his distress warrants loving responses. This relationship creates in the child a healthy superego because it builds a positive self-concept, positive relationships, and healthy boundaries between self and others. Children with healthy superegos seem to effortlessly master life's developmental challenges without succumbing to victimization, or to bullying others. (Sroufe, 2005) As adults, they are resilient and have the opportunity to live rewarding lives. Their superego promotes adaptive behaviors. Most importantly, affirming Freud's belief that children absorb the unconscious part of the parent's superego, they seem to pass these gifts on to their children. (Main, 2000)

The secure conditions described above are seen in about 50–60% of the world's population. (van IJzendoorn, 2008) The remaining 40–50% are less fortunate. (Sroufe, 2005) These children have caregivers who are some combination of rejecting, emotionally shut down, dismissive, devaluing, critical, or aggressive; they lack attunement and perhaps have faulty—or intrusive—boundaries. These children associate distress with unloving responses. These children's superegos take the form of their uncaring aggressor, whether that lack of care was through overt hostility or through covert acts of neglect. This internalized aggressor is encoded in the child's brain for life, and affects his or her functioning throughout the life cycle. This influence has been referred to as "Ghosts from the Nursery." (Karen-Morse, R, 1997)

As we said earlier, attachment is the necessary matrix for the child's attachment bond. Attachment, however, is not merely a psychological phenomenon; it is also a neurobiological process that is crucial to the development of a healthy mind, brain, body, and relationships. The attachment relationship gives form and structure to the way in which the most primitive parts of the brain develop. To us it is self-evident that the child initially sees itself through the eyes of its attachment figure. We hypothesize that it is primarily through the brain's mirror neuronal system (among others) that the child internalizes his attachment figure's view of himself: he sees himself as if through the caregiver's eyes.

Researchers are only beginning to understand the power and influence of the mirror neuronal system, but our clinical experience supports the notion that this system reflects the way in which the attachment figure treats the child.

Discovery of Mirror Neurons

A mirror neuron is a neuron that fires both when an animal acts and when the animal observes the same action performed by another (Rizzolatti, et al,

2004). Thus, the neuron "mirrors" the behavior of the other, as though the observer himself were acting.[1]

The function of the mirror system is a subject of much speculation,[2] but there is compelling, albeit inferential, evidence for the mirror neuron systems involvement in empathy, and thus superego development (Preston and Frans de Waal, 2002; Decety, 2002, 2004; Gallese, 1998,

---

1. Such neurons have been directly observed in primates, and are believed to occur in humans. In humans, brain activity consistent with that of mirror neurons has been found in the premotor cortex and the inferior parietal cortex, and some researchers believe they might be part of the process of imitation and language acquisition (Ramachandran, 2006). However, prior to this paper, no widely accepted neural or computational models have been put forward to describe how mirror neuron activity supports cognitive functions such as imitation.

2. Mirror systems may simulate observed actions, and thus contribute to theory of mind skills (Keysers, 2006; Arbib, 2004). They may also be related to language abilities. (Hugo, 2002) Approximately 10% of neurons in a monkey's inferior frontal and inferior parietal cortex have 'mirror' properties and give similar responses to performed hand actions and to observed actions. In both humans and monkeys the mirror system also responds to the sound of actions (Keysers, 2006). Mirror neurons have been found in both inferior frontal (Kilner, 2009) and inferior parietal regions of the brain. (Gallesse, 1996; Fogassi, 2005) Evidence from functional neuroimaging and behavioral neuroimaging strongly suggests the presence of similar mirror neurons systems in humans.

Functional magnetic resonance imaging indicates that a much wider network of brain areas shows mirror properties in humans than previously thought. These additional areas include the somatosensory cortex, the inferior frontal cortex and the superior parietal lobe. There brain regions have been defined as the human mirror neuron system. (Iacoboni, 1999) The pattern of activity in these brain regions is similar during the perception of other people's actions and while performing similar actions, which supports the notion of a human mirror neuron system. (Etzel, 2008, Dinstien 2007).

Several indirect measures have been used to study the mirror neuron system in humans. For example, when a person observes another person's action, his motor cortex becomes ready to discharge. (Fadiga, 1999) Studies have linked mirror neurons to our capability to understand other people's goals and intentions.

2001).[3] Experiments have shown that certain brain regions (in particular the anterior insula, anterior cingulate cortex, and inferior frontal cortex) are active when a person experiences an emotion (disgust, happiness, pain, etc.), as well as when he or she sees another person experiencing an emotion. (Botvinik, 2005; Lamm, 2007) However, these brain regions are not quite the same as the ones which mirror hand actions. Mirror neurons for emotional states or empathy have not yet been described in monkeys; therefore, much of our current understanding is simply speculation. And yet it has also been demonstrated that people who are more empathic according to self-report questionnaires have stronger activations both in the mirror system for hand actions (Singer, 2004) and the mirror system for emotions, providing more direct support for the idea that the mirror system is linked to empathy. (Keysers, 2007)

Empathy Linked with Guilt

The underpinning of primitive pre-verbal guilt is the capacity to understand that others have the same feelings and longings as we ourselves do. The mirror neuron system supplies a theoretical basis wherein an infant can feel pain over the harm it imagines that it did to its caregiver. Davanloo's system of therapy sees unconscious empathy-guilt capacity as the platform upon which the Punitive Superego is constructed. A mature superego will encourage undoing behavior or thoughts as the adaptive response to hurtful behavior; the immature superego demands suffering to repair the guilt.

Theory of Mind

"Theory of Mind" refers to our ability to infer another person's mental state (*i.e.,* beliefs and desires) from their experiences or their behavior. (Baron-Cohen, 2001) For example, if you see a child reaching into a jar labeled 'cookies,' you might assume that she wants a cookie (even if you know the jar is empty). In many ways "Theory of Mind" describes the

---

3. The superego's evolutionary adaptive advantage is that it controls intra-familial aggressive behavior.

mechanism of projection and makes it a normal psychic process. It is easy to see how this normal process has adaptive value in being able to read the intentions of others. It seems self-evident that if this process is not checked with reality testing it becomes the basis of all self-referential thinking.[4] Consequently, there is a continuum from empathy to guilt, as well as from empathy to paranoia.

There are several competing models that attempt to account for Theory of Mind. The most notable in relation to mirror neurons is simulation theory. According to simulation theory, we subconsciously empathize with the person we're observing and, accounting for relevant differences, imagine what we would desire and believe in that scenario. (Goldman, A., 1989; Gallese, V., Goldman, A., 1998) Mirror neurons are thought to be essential in developing a mental representation not only of the other's mental and emotional state, but also of their intentions. (Schulte-Ruther, M, et al; Gallese, V, Goldman, A.)

This is a highly complex process composed, in part, of intelligence, projection, reality testing and empathy. Therefore, we believe it is reasonable to assume that a child internalizes the attachment pattern of his caretaker through this mechanism and builds the parent's mind side by side with his own experiential self as an observer and judge of all his feelings. It is of clinical importance for AB-ISTDP that it is the actual contingent harmful interaction between child and caregiver is both the trigger for the mobilization of unconscious rage, guilt and grief and the source of superego pathology. We believe that there is an inherent archetypal drive towards secure attachment which, when thwarted, predisposes a child toward the development of a Punitive Superego. Most importantly, even if it is not the caregiver who thwarts the attachment, the caregiver still becomes the object of the unconscious rage for the implied failure to protect the child from harm. (See discussion on double PI below.)

---

4. As this system is being laid down, between six and eighteen months of life, the capacity for reality testing is limited, and it is only when the left hemisphere (along with the older right hemisphere) matures, that reality testing can be effective as a check and balance to faulty assumptions.

Punitive Superego and Psychopathology

Once internalized, as outlined above, the Punitive Superego becomes embedded with the entire process of instinctual gratification and need satisfaction. It is a force which then sustains and rewards maladaptive functioning.

Common Presentations of Projective Identification

Projective Identification, as we have outlined above, is an intra- and inter-psychic phenomena which deserves a clinician's careful study. Even in its most obvious manifestation, it is a complex process. Davanloo distinguishes projective identification, double projective identification and multiple projective identification. Still, the question arises whether this distinction is useful. A patient normally will use his specific defense repertoire in his several interactions. If a patient identifies, projects, splits, intellectualizes, etc., he will bring these defenses into operation in his several interactions. We don't speak of identification, double identification, multiple identification. Therefore, this distinction seems unnecessary. (oral communication with Josette ten Have-de Labije, 2008)

Single Projective Identification

Bill is a man in late middle age in an unhappy relationship with a girlfriend with whom he is in conflict over how she relates to her son. His relationship was one of caretaking for his partner instead of passion and love. He saw the therapist to find out why he was so unhappy, and wanted to commit to a genuine loving relationship.

We did a successful trial therapy and what emerged during the first unlocking of his unconscious (when the complex transference feelings were mobilized) was acute pain in his right shoulder. The pain was unbearable, searing and sharp. His anxiety pathway was entirely striated muscle and he was poised for a breakthrough. He imagined shooting me as an expression of his rage. This aggravated his shoulder pain. Guilt and grief over my shooting followed along with the visual image of him aiming his father's gun at his older brother (his father's favorite), deciding to kill him and pulling the trigger. The pain in his shoulder became unbearable in intensity. Bill recovered the actual image of the bullet entering his beagle dog's shoulder that happened to be sitting on his brother's lap at the time he pulled the trigger. He felt profound guilt towards the dog as well as his brother and parents for the pain he wanted and did inflict on them. He cried profusely over his loss of attachment security after the guilt passed. He saw the link with his jealousy of his girlfriend. He never felt shoulder pain again after the trial therapy.

Discussion

Bill was rivalrous with his brother and angry with his father for favoring his brother. He acted out his impulse to kill his brother but accidentally shot his dog. Bill had repressed the whole painful experience, but chose to punish himself with chronic and acute shoulder pain and a loveless life. His rage had hurt his dog's shoulder and his mirror neuronal system identified with the victim of his rage—his brother and his dog. When he visualized the dog being shot he had a major unlocking of guilt and grief and the patient's more mature ego was able forgive himself rather than punish himself.

Double Projective Identification

Daniel was a brilliant Harvard graduate who never filled his potential in business. He sought therapy for a phobia of success, as well as an unhappy marital stalemate with unsatisfactory intimacy. During a series of block therapy treatments, he developed right buttock pain with no medical cause.

Historically Daniel was close to his mother who was warm, loving and empathic. His father was domineering, possessive and devaluing. Whenever he was with Daniel's mother Daniel was made an outsider as his father refused to share his wife's warmth with Daniel. Daniel's mother was compliant and accepted this situation. At age 16 she developed terminal cancer and he was excluded from any grief goodbye process—his father again subordinated him.

During his unlocking he developed the false belief that he was anally sodomized by his father. With further unlocking he envisioned two destructive images: painfully killing his father with a pole inserted in his anus and murdering and (anally) raping his mother for her submission to his father's instructions. With the passage of these images he became pain-free. As a result, he stopped punishing his wife by creating distance between them and by subordinating her to his daughter.

Discussion

Daniel internalized the pain that he imagined inflicting on his father and mother; the closer he would get to his complex transference feelings, the more the pain would intensify. Allowing the visualization of the unconscious image into consciousness removed the physical pain. Once the repressed action tendency was felt and then visualized to completion, along with an experience of guilt and grief, the somatic reactivity is permanently removed, and adaptive flexibility restored. Once again, the mirror neuron system is "reprogrammed." Since we are frequently enraged by the same stimulus and even unconsciously reshape relationships to produce similar situations to feel enraged in, the cycle of trauma, rage, guilt and self-punishment becomes recursive. It is our belief that the neuronal circuit underlying this process increases in density and the need for revenge and punishment grows progressively more powerful—perhaps insatiable.

The Man with the Ghost in the Basement and in the Nursery

The following is an annotated case example of eight hours of a total seventeen-hour block treatment. It demonstrates separating ego from superego (ten Have-de Labije, 2009), followed by undoing the effects of projective identification.

Phase One: Separating the Punitive Superego from the Ego

Day One: The patient is a forty-nine-year-old recently married man who lives in California. His wife of two years, Michelle, is pregnant with twins. She miscarried a previous pregnancy. His history is notable for the chronic ego-syntonic use of alcohol, marijuana and cocaine. He has been in therapy with various practitioners for twenty years and was referred to Dr. Neborsky by his marriage therapist to address the verbally abusive fighting between him and his wife.

When the patient was ten years old, his twenty-one-year-old brother Rick hung himself in the basement of the family home. The patient has just finished describing a heated argument he recently had with his wife. He characterized the argument as a "blow-up" which he "wanted to stop." We start the transcript one hour into the session. The therapist begins with inquiry.

T: Why couldn't you disengage, why couldn't you stop?
P: I couldn't stop.
T: Why?
P: I don't know.
T: Think about it: what was driving your behavior? You don't have self-control?
P: It doesn't feel like I have self-control.
T: Oh, that's a problem.
P: I agree it is a problem.
T: How old are you?
P: I will be forty-nine.
T: Well, just a take a look back. How has a lack of self-control harmed you?
P: Well, I guess doing drugs all those years. You know from fourteen until now—even though I don't perceive it as harming me, it has harmed me. I don't think that my memory is as good; I think I may have achieved more in life. Maybe I would have had better . . . I've isolated my entire life.
T: Do you remember jumping off the roof?

Earlier, the patient told the therapist that once, while intoxicated, he jumped from a roof.

P: I remember jumping off the roof.
T: You almost killed yourself.
P: Close to it. I didn't stop, though. I just continued to party after that. Even though I broke my teeth. It didn't matter to me.
T: So it's stunning to me that you don't recognize yourself as a person with poor impulse control . . . It's stunning.
P: Well yeah, it is stunning. It is stunning.
T: You started commenting about something to me, something about anxiety. I didn't mean to shut you up.

P: No, no, you were following another thought.
T: No, they are all related, aren't they.
P: Yeah, I think so, absolutely.
T: Why do you suffer from anxiety?
P: I have been wondering about that a lot—why I am an anxious person.

The psychotherapist is subtly confronting the patient's denial, rationalization, and minimization of his self-destructive resistance.

The patient reveals that his mother gave birth to a son in a previous marriage. In a terrible accident, she dropped the infant, and he died. She divorced, married the patient's father, and gave birth to him. The therapist asks him to imagine what his mother felt when he was born.

P: I could only imagine the guilt, the suffering, and the anxiety not to drop me. "Don't drop the baby," so to speak.
T: "Don't kill another baby . . ."

The psychotherapist is mirroring the maternal superego showing empathy as if the patient is being viewed with the mother's eyes.

P: Don't kill another baby, exactly. I think I was constantly paid attention to. I was never left alone. I remember being in the bathroom . . . there was never a private moment. I was always with my mother. Then when I had to separate from my mother, I was incredibly anxious. I didn't want to go anywhere without my mother. I didn't want to be anywhere. . . . When I had to get in my first carpool, I kicked and screamed and cried and did whatever I could not to get in that other car.
T: So you were having separation anxiety.
P: Absolutely. I think this anxiety from childhood has been my anxiety throughout life. Now after a certain age I probably got. . . . I never did like birthday parties. I never enjoyed them or my birthday per se. I got over that and I was fine and it seemed that we were fine as a family. Up until Rick killed himself.

The patient reveals that when his mother found his brother hanging in the basement she was "incredibly calm." She brought the patient to his aunt's house where he was given a Valium. The therapist asks if this was his first expe-

rience with drugs-as-comfort. The patient recalls that at the age of six, his parents gave him small liquor bottles to play with, and he got "wildly drunk." His parents took the bottles from him. He told them, "If you won't let me have the little bottles, then I'll drink from the big bottles." The therapist observes that the patient doesn't take "No" for an answer, and that when he wants something, he gets it, even if that something could harm him. Subsequently, the therapist asks him if he think he has a chemical dependency disorder.

P: Actually, I don't. I actually think that it's naïve for me to say that, but I don't think of myself as having a chemical dependency disorder.

T: Why do you say that it is naïve for you to think that?

P: Because I've used chemicals my whole life and I've been attracted to them and they've been a part of my existence.

The psychotherapist confronts of the patient's denial of his problems with substances, acting out, and treatment resistance.

T: But then again I don't know who I'm talking to because you have fluctuating states of mind. On the one hand you say, "No, I don't really think that way about myself," and then on the other you say, "Yes, I do think that way about myself." So which of these two people do I believe? You seem to be describing to me in very clear terms, in very black and very white terms, all the problems associated with having a personality disorder.

P: Yeah.

T: Do you see what I'm saying?

P: Yes, I can understand yes.

T: Right. In other words, you have an inability to delay gratification of impulses; you have free-floating anxiety; you have low frustration tolerance. You act out to alleviate your immediate distress, irrespective of long term consequences.

P: Right.

T: So, conclusion . . . ?

P: That I have a chemical . . . not dependency but a . . .

T: No dependency. You're not addicted; you're dependent upon mood-altering substances and mood-altering responses from people.

P: Yes.

T: You have an immature kind of "weak ego."

P: Right. Intellectually, I can understand what you are saying, but—

T: Yeah, that's where we start, intellectually.

P: But for me to embody, you know . . . I don't want to. I don't want to think that I have a weak ego, or I have some lame duck as part of my personality. I don't like it and I don't want to hold that.

T: But again, isn't this now the immature ego talking, because what does this insight produce inside of you? What's your reaction to this insight that I am sharing with you? Your reaction to it?

P: My reaction to it is to fight it.

T: No, that's your defense mechanism. I'm asking you what is the emotion that this intellectual input is creating inside of you. What is the feeling response inside that you're defending against as you're sitting here with me?

P: It makes me feel fearful; it's scary to me. I have this (patient takes deep breath) feeling like in my gut . . .

T: You're having anxiety.

P: Anxiety, yes.

T: OK, good. Now here is where you're screwed. OK? Because you have the fear response in the wrong place. OK? The way you approach your life is what's scary. Your self-destructive personality. So you decide which part of you is the part that you want to ally with and which part you want to overcome.

The patient reacts to this confrontation with a series of intellectual defenses and projections. The therapist identifies and challenges these defenses while pressuring the patient to feel his emotions. We are ninety minutes into the session.

T: So you can see the part of you, the immature part of you, just keeps putting up with defenses?

P: Right.

T: Because you don't want to feel this feeling of anxiety and emotion about your chronic habitual self-destructive treatment. You know, immature, self-destructive treatment of yourself.

P: No I don't.

T: You would rather go jumping from the frying pan into fire, like you've done your entire life?

P: Right.

T: So which is it going to be? Are you going to address your feelings or are you going to escape from them?

P: I want to address them.

T: Fabulous, let's do it. What's the feeling down there that's making you sick to your stomach? You said there's a part of it that is anxiety. If you look at it like this, this is your feeling part; this is your anxiety part; the feeling of anxiety since your childhood. . . . The earliest part of your childhood put a lid on your feeling part, it capped it.

P: Yes.

T: OK. What you have described to me was when you wanted to separate from your mother you couldn't do it because you became crippled by overwhelming anxiety.

P: Right.

T: So you never learned to regulate your anxiety on your own behalf.

P: Right.

T: You were a victim of your own anxiety; you never learned the techniques or the strategies to regulate your anxieties. Hence, you have become an addictive personality. You are always looking for environmental things to make you feel better.

P: Right.

T: That's not autonomy. That's not self-regulation. That's being an environmentally dependent human being.

P: Right.

T: How long have you suffered from this?

P: It's frightening for me, it's very frightening, you know. I've just *(takes deep breath)* . . . It's not what I want. It's certainly very uncomfortable.

T: So you are not happy right now?

P: I'm. . . .

T: I'm serious when I say that.

P: I'm happy in a sense that I enjoy understanding . . . I'm enjoying the fact that you are reaching me and that this is actually . . . I'm following you. So there is a happiness that—thank God—that something is happening.

T: Good.

P: But. . . .

T: What are you unhappy about?

P: I am very sad that I did not acquire the skills in life and that I have had to medicate and have my environment create who I am instead of having me create who I am.

T: How sad is your life actually when you look at it through this lens?

P: I wish I could say that it is sad enough; I wish I could say that it is so sad that I can't continue. . . .

T: I just said how sad is it?

P: Right.

T: Come on now, don't bullshit me.

P: I'm not bullshitting you. I'm saying that I'm not that—

T: You're saying that I wish I could say . . .

P: I wish I could say that I am oh-so-sad that—

T: I wish you could say what is accurate. How sad are you?

P: I'm not that sad.

T: OK, could we take a look at your deceased brother. You never got to see him did you?

P: No.

T: But you imagined him, right?

P: Yes.

The therapist asks the patient to express his true feelings about his brother's suicide. After some resistance, the patient says he feels anger at his brother for being his role model in self-destruction. The therapist reviews the patient's childhood traumas and notes that he seems to lack any compassion for himself.

T: Do you understand what I am saying?

P: Yes.

T: What's your reaction to it?

P: I want to examine this. I want to see why.

T: That's lip service. What is your reaction, your gut, gut, gut . . .

P: Gut is right.

T: Fine. I'm right. There are plenty of psychotherapists who are right. Your reaction in your gut—what is your feeling inside?

P: The feeling. . . .

T: Happy, sad, glad . . . ?

P: No sad, sad. This is actually the first sadness that I've felt towards myself.

From our point of view, the patient was entirely identified with his unhealthy punitive superego. He had been following the dictates of his punitive side (the dictates of his internalized mother: deny and/or devalue your longings, feelings, autonomy, strength in order to make up for my guilt) for most of his life and was devoid of insight into his self-destructive actions. The first session was two hours of confrontation with, identification and clarification of his detached and uninvolved stance toward his longings, feelings, problems. At no point was the therapist willing to engage with the patient's detached and denying stance towards his emotions, longings and problems until the patient created a meaningful separation from his denying, minimizing, and detaching punitive superego.

Phase 2: Restructuring Ego-Adaptive Capacity and Exploration of the Triangles of Conflict and Persons

Day Two: The patient thinks about yesterday's session, and finds he agrees with much of what the therapist said. He admits to having an immature ego and that he is accustomed to instant gratification.

He also finds himself devaluing the therapist and doubting the validity of what he said. He bridles at the idea that his "self-destructiveness" is "abundantly clear."

The therapist observes that the patient has a pattern of verbally attacking (devaluing and putting at doubt) those who don't mirror his own state of mind. The therapist points out that the patient cannot delay gratification of an impulse because he was never taught how to manage his anxiety nor his feelings as a child.

The patient admits feeling anxiety at this very moment and clearly observes his physical symptoms. He also observes that underneath his anxiety he feels anger towards the therapist.

Now that the patient has separated his healthy desire for secure attachment from his unhealthy part (identification with the dictate of his superego), it is possible to examine the state of his ego-adaptive capacity and his feelings through the lens of the triangle of conflict. We are one hour into the session.

T: So what are the feelings underneath your anxiety, if you don't revert to old behavior? Old behavior being ignoring, lying, being sloppy, or being lazy. (his self-defeating defenses)

P: I'm not sure about feeling anger because I am still feeling anxious.

T: Excellent, excellent observing, excellent . . . go on. Understand that the anxiety is crippling your force.

P: I do understand; it is making me tired, making me drowsy.

T: You are still cutting off the aggression with anxiety. Is that what you want to do? Do you want to cut off your anxiety with aggression? You have done this your whole life.

P: Right.

T: Do you want to do this?

P: No.

T: OK, what do you want to do?

P: I want to release my anxiety.

T: OK, but how? You're observing it.

P: Yes, observing.

T: But what do you also have to observe?

P: The other things that prolong anxiety.

T: That are creating the anxiety. The aggression is creating the anxiety. You said that when you get aggressive that you have learned to go into an altered state of consciousness. You go into some dreamlike state.

P: Even when I was aggressive, um, towards you, when I wasn't here, it made me very tired.

T: OK, tell me about that aggression towards me.

P: When I was discussing what had gone here yesterday with Michelle.

T: Yeah.

P: It made me really tired and sleepy.

T: OK, but tell me about the aggression, not the anxiety. Remember, getting tired and sleepy is you going into a coma.

The patient is unable to distinguish impulse (aggression) from anxiety and his defense of dissociation. This confirmed the psychotherapist's suspicion that the patient has low ego-adaptive capacity.

P: Right, it's the—

T: It's the opposite of aggression.

P: Right, right, it's the opposite.

T: It's the opposite of aggression. Can you be aggressive? Can you be an aggressive person, yes or no?

P: Yes.

T: Right, so you are doing everything in your power right now to subdue your aggression, and I am trying to point out to you that some of the things that you are doing to subdue your aggression are unhealthy for your long-term well being. But you are holding onto it as if it were a valuable thing to do, like comas are a good thing. Do you want to live your life comatose?

P: No, that is what I have been doing. I have been living my whole life comatose.

T: I know you have. So wake up and feel your aggression. You said that you were aggressive to me when you talked to your wife. What was that like?

P: The aggressive part was to destroy.

T: I understand. But describe . . . carefully.

P: Feels almost like a tornado, like, um . . . spun out of control.

T: Huge amount of force.

P: Huge amount of force. Like if I could have fire-bombed this office last night, if I could have terrorized you somehow, um—

T: OK, but that's a bit indirect. What if that force were released against me directly?

P: The actual anger or the actual aggression?

T: Yeah. You said you would want, or it would give you to a certain degree satisfaction, to destroy me.

P: Right.

T: And how would you do that? How would you destroy me?

P: I think that I would physically want to tear you apart.

T: OK.

P: Physically, get into it with you, even if I had to potentially get hurt myself.

T: OK, I understand. Do you have a mental image on your mind of that?

P: I do.

T: That's good. And what do you see in that image?

P: I see physical violence between the two of us. I see us physically fighting and tearing at each other.

T: OK, but I am most interested in your part. What would you physically be doing to me? Tearing at me, how would you be tearing at me in that image? What would be your goal?

P: Punching you, pulling your hair, scratching you, biting you, destroying and poking your eyes out, destroying your sight, pulling your limbs off your body, ravaging, you know, ripping your insides out.

T: So I would be mauled.

P: Yes.

T: Just mauled. And at a certain point, is there a relief that you experience?

P: No.

T: Why not?

P: Because I am still enraged.

T: There is more that you would like to destroy.

P: It almost feels like . . . it doesn't feel like there was a stop to it. It doesn't even feel like when you are destroyed, and I have tasted your blood and I have bitten you in half, I don't feel . . . *(sigh)*

T: There is a lot happening inside, there was a . . . I saw a *(sigh, takes deep breath)* there's a rising of significant amount of feelings.

P: I still feel there is more to destroy.

T: I understand. But there were other things that happened in your mind. What were the other things that happened? There was a rise there for a moment of energy.

P: I took it away from you for moment and took it to my wife.

T: What were the pictures that flashed into your mind?

P: I was trying to destroy her and the children; I was stomping on her stomach, killing the children, making her suffer.

T: And you receive a certain degree of satisfaction at that point?

P: I did. I felt free. I felt that even though I'm not sure of what my consequences were I felt—

T: Don't worry about consequences, it's silly. This is imagery.

P: It felt like once I was able to destroy, once my aggression was able to destroy . . .

T: Destroy the life in her belly.

P: The children—destroy their life and rip them from her. Then I'm free of her.

T: Yeah, it's hard for me to tell but it seems that she does not survive either.

P: She does survive.

T: She does survive, and that's what you want? To just destroy the two children and to make her suffer a great deal of physical and, I imagine, emotional pain?

P: Yes.

T: And that gave you satisfaction and relief?

P: Yes, and relief.

T: And are there actual fetuses that you see that you destroyed?

P: No, because they are completely mauled and I don't really see, you know.

T: That is fine, what you see is what you see.

P: Now I can tell you that I am going back to anxiety again.

T: You did go back to anxiety.

P: Absolutely.

T: Describe it please.

P: Extreme dizziness.

T: You had an extreme spike of dizziness.

P: Extreme spike of dizziness, extreme spike of tension, dry mouth.

T: OK, alright. So you understand now, the function of anxiety is to suppress your deeper register of emotions. The first emotion that we examined here is sadness. You know, you felt a sadness that you were not able to connect to me in the way that you wanted to connect. The next emotion that we had to work to get to was an aggressive emotion with a certain degree of cruelty and a desire to hurt, not just to destroy, but to hurt. So there were two components to the destruction: one was towards the children, another component of the destruction was towards Michelle. Then when you allowed that to sink in, that gave you relief, and that is when the anxiety spiked. I am very interested in what you're feeling that is making you so massively anxious. And I wish that you wouldn't block yourself.

At the moment when the patient is about to experience his guilt, he exceeds his processing capacity so the therapist backs off and summarizes the process to strengthen the patient's ego-adaptive capacity.

P: It feels like despair. After all the carnage is done, and after everything, and after I have destroyed the babies and my wife, the first feeling is release and the second feeling is despair.

T: Oh, OK. Is the anxiety feeling a little lower?

P: Yes.

T: Well done. So just let yourself feel that despair. Don't try to escape from it. Anything you can tell me about it would be enormously helpful to you, not just in here, but in your life out there. Anything you can tell me about your despair . . . is there a picture in your mind?

P: A picture? I see my wife's body destroyed and I see parts of her insides and outside. I don't see the children but I know that they are dead and the despair is that I know that I can't fix this, I can't change this ever. This is now. This is forever. I have killed my children. I have destroyed my wife.

T: Maimed her. She is not dead.

P: She is not dead but she is severely hurt. She will never be the same.

T: So if I am reading your face, it is kind of a sad regretful experience, is that . . .

P: Yes, and for the little bit of relief that I got and after knowing that I was released, the despair is that I have to live with knowing what I have done. I cannot bear to look at what I have done.

Again the patient nears his experiential threshold and he avoids the painful emotion of guilt over the destruction of the two children and his wife. The therapist will help the patient to bear and contain his guilt by inviting him to look into his wife's eyes.

T: So again there is more emotion over what you have done. What is the emotion when you look at what you have done? Only look at what you have done, what is the feeling?

P: It makes me feel sick.

T: Nausea-sick or a different sick?

P: It is a nausea-sick feeling.

T: The anxiety keeps spiking.

P: Yes.

T: What I would like to ask you to do is, to actually approach your wife, not walk away from, but to actually look into her eyes and tell me what you see.

P: She won't look at me. She can look at me, but she won't look at me.

T: But you can see.

P: I can look into her eyes.

T: OK, good.

P: She can physically have her eyes cast upon me but there is nothing there looking at me.

T: But you can see.

P: I can see her

T: And are you able to describe to me with precision again the color of eyes, not what you think the color is by knowing.

P: They are a cold, cold gray.

T: You actually see, you see grayness.

P: I see grayness.

T: And it seems to be anxiety-provoking for you if I am seeing your face accurately. Is there a bit of anxiety?

P: Yes.

T: So let's please intervene on the anxiety because it is too important for you. Because I would like you to look at her eyes with a tad, just a tad of curiosity. OK? And allow a color to appear in her irises, just allow those eyes to have a color in them without making a conscious decision as to whose eyes you see. Just let it happen.

P: They are green.

T: And I can observe a rise of emotion in your throat when you said green. There seems to be significance to the greenness.

P: My mother's eyes were green.

The patient describes visualizing his mother as physically intact, but emotionally vacant. The therapist suggests that as a child this would have been sad for him since we are genetically programmed to want to make our mothers happy. This concept produces another spike of anxiety in the patient. We are two hours into the session.

P: Wow.

T: What is coming up?

P: I want to grieve, I want the grief to come out and every time I want to let it come out, I mask it with my anxiety.

T: What do you have to grieve over?

P: I have grief over not making my mother happy.

T: And why couldn't you make your mother happy?

P: Because she's already sad and depressed and there is nothing I could do. I see myself reaching towards her face, I see my hand reaching towards her face to touch her face, then pulling back, crying a tear, not being there with me, not acknowledging my touch.

T: And what does that feel like inside?

P: I feel like I have been a tragic person. There is such a disproportionate sadness. I don't carry a lot of happiness and am not free.

Dr. Neborsky asks the patient to complete his murderous fantasy and to tell how he would bury his "murdered" children. We are two-and-a-half hours into the session.

P: I see that I would have to embrace them and hold them and look at what I have done to them. I would have to kiss them and find a beautiful place for them to be and rest and I just can't let them go and I just think, I push the dirt just so slowly, so, so slowly. I just push a little bit and I just get a small, small handful and I just very slowly cover them.

The therapist helps the patient understand that his rage towards his mother gets evoked in relationships with anyone who gets close to him, even to his own unborn children (onto whom he projects himself). The patient's guilt and grief over this unconscious murderous rage has caused him to lead a life of emotional isolation, and to self-medicate. The patient then reports back about the session, comparing what he felt last night to what he feels at the present moment.

P: Yesterday I was stunned, in a way, that there was aggression towards you. Today I am stunned in a way . . . it's stunning to hear these things and to accept them and to know that they are true. I think this is exactly what I have been striving for and I do not want my life to be a tragedy.

Psychodynamically, the patient's unconscious had carried his mother's unresolved bereavement over the death of her two children. Her projective identification of her two "murdered children" was too heavy for her to carry so my patient absorbed the weight of her guilt. When he fell in love with his wife he had no idea what a time bomb lurked within.

By chance or destiny, the fact that his wife was carrying twins was overwhelming to him. He could not allow himself (identification with his internalized mother) to love two children (projection of himself and of his brother he had to replace) since she (and because of the patient's identification with his internalized mother) was responsible for the death of two of her children.

Her unresolved depression caused him to feel both unloved and over-protected (undermining of autonomy) and he had unconscious rage towards her for her emotional neglect of him. The undoing of the patient's projective identification, mobilization and conscious experience of his rage, guilt and grief towards his mother gave him a new chance to positively identify with his loving father. This takes place in Phase 3.

Phase 3: Restoration of the Healthy Superego

Day Three: The patient talks about how much he adored his father, but admits that he "wasn't there for him" during his father's long hospital stay, having visited him only once. Dr. Neborsky asks why this is so. The patient responds with vagueness, finally admitting that he was furious at the doctors who diagnosed his father's illness. Dr. Neborsky asks who became the real victim of his rage. The patient says that <u>he</u> became the victim of his own rage. Dr. Neborsky asks the patient to describe his last meeting with his father. We are one hour and forty-five minutes into the session.

T: So again, tell me when was the last time you saw your father alive?

P: It was in the hospital. He was smiling, he was always happy to see me. I don't know the exact last time but he would always put on a happy face. His gut reaction every time he saw me was to smile and to be cheerful and he would sing and act as if he didn't have a care in the world.

T: But the key question that I have for you is, what did you leave unsaid, unspoken? What do you regret?

P: This is a nightmare for me, a nightmare to see my father.

T: What are the feelings associated with being in a nightmare?

P: Anger. I wanted to kill everyone in the hospital, I wanted to kill all the nurses and the staff, I wanted to come down with a machine gun and kill them all.

T: So that is just profound rage.

P: I wanted to kill their families; I wanted to make them suffer.

T: Profound rage. Is there more that the rage wants to do?

P: The anxiety is coming again.

T: OK, and could you give me information about your state of mind? What's going on inside when you hear my words?

P: Like television, I feel really far away.

T: Oh, OK. So the anxiety is in your thinking process. Now I am just going to ask a question. . . . In you is there a judgment going on about that killing spree? How many people do you think that you have murdered in that fantasy? How many?

P: Hundreds. As many as I could, before I get killed . . . before they kill me.

T: OK, this is what they call "suicide by cop." Have you ever heard that expression?

P: No.

T: You have never heard that expression "suicide by cop"?

P: Oh, OK, now I got you.

T: See there was another part to the fantasy that never got. . . .

P: That I feel the same death that my father is feeling, that I experience death with him.

T: Do you see that you did not want to separate from your father?

P: Yes.

T: That it was unbearable to you? Now is this new knowledge for you?

P: Yes.

T: Is it of value to you?

P: Yes.

T: Tell me the value it has to you.

P: I thought I separated from my father long before. I didn't know that I was still connected with him. I thought that we were so different; we had different interests . . . that we weren't close.

T: What is so clear to me is that you don't want to say goodbye to your father. You don't want to do it. It's too painful. So you would rather suffer than say goodbye. You seem to be reacting to my words.

P: I was reacting to the anxiety.

T: What was the reacting?

P: The reacting at first was, I was thinking about the unconditional relationship of dad. I was thinking about how back when I was an infant, I would smile at him and he would smile back at me. When I looked into my father's eyes there was love.

Dr. Neborsky notes that over and over again the patient describes his father as a man who was always emotionally available. He then asks the patient to describe his father's funeral. We are two hours and fifteen minutes into the session.

T: Tell me about the funeral.

P: I got there and I was on either Ativan or I was on Valium or some kind of sedative and I had not gotten there days before that to see him, I think. . . . I don't know if he was buried the next day or if it was the day in between or. . . .

T: Whoa, whoa, whoa, whoa, why did you tell me that?

P: Because I didn't get there soon enough, I got there the day of the funeral.

T: Why did you tell me that? What is the emotion?

P: Being ashamed, because I should have gotten here sooner.

T: That's a defense.

P: Anger.

The patient again defends against feelings of guilt.

T: No, guilt.

P: Oh.

T: That's a healthy part of you that feels guilty, don't punish yourself, your father would not . . .

P: He would not punish me.

T: He would not be happy. What would he say to you? If his spirit were sitting here, what would he say to you?

P: He would say . . . let me go, it's OK. Let me go.

T: Would he be happy if he knew that you planned to punish yourself to eternity?

P: No.

T: What would he say?

P: He would say you have to be a man now; you have to take care of your wife and your children.

T: Instead of what?

P: Instead of being the child.

T: And driving her away?

P: And driving her away, and he would want me to be like him, a loving father.

T: You seem deeply connected to your love of your father right now. It's a good feeling in a way, isn't it? He was a very compassionate human being. He didn't believe in punishment as a virtue.

P: No, no, he was always kind.

T: So again, take me back to the actual funeral again. Where did you sit?

P: I wanted to see him before the funeral, so I went into the room where the casket was and I was really surprised to see that it was an ornate casket. Because I thought my grandmother's funeral was the only funeral that I had ever been to, and her casket was just a pine box. It was a kosher casket—it was just pine and it had a Jewish star on it and it wasn't supposed to have any nails; there is not supposed to be any metal if it is kosher. There is not to be any metal. So when I saw my father's casket it seemed shiny and ornate a little bit and I thought I don't understand this. I didn't understand why he wasn't in a pine box. I am sure my father would want to be buried in a kosher casket and I was confused and then . . . Ummm, I opened the casket and I saw my father there and I touched his skin and he was cold. I kissed him a couple of times and I just kept my lips on his cheek.

T: And you are letting yourself feel the love.

P: I feel the love of my father and I was the only one in the room. The funeral director came in and told me that it was time and that I had to go out. I said no I needed more time, don't do it now. He said no that I had to do it now, and then I screamed at him.

T: So you didn't want to part.

P: I didn't want to part.

T: I understand.

P: I said I needed more time, give me more time, give me a few more minutes . . . Five more minutes. He didn't want to do it and I told him just to get out, I'm taking it anyway.

T: So you were ferocious.

P: I was.

T: You were ferocious standing up for your time with your father.

P: And finally he came back and then I said OK.

T: And what was that like when you and he parted.

P: My father and I?

T: Yes . . . you said OK.

P: I am not sure, I don't remember.

T: Picture it, how did you part? You said you were kissing him.

P: I closed the . . .

T: You closed the casket.

P: I kissed him one more time; I kissed him on the lips.

T: And what were your goodbye words? Even if you didn't express them at the time.

P: I'm sorry. I'm sorry I wasn't there for you. I love you.

T: And did you ask him for forgiveness?

P: No.

T: And if you had, what would you say? About you not being there for him?

P: He would say, "I would always forgive you, son. I would always forgive you."

T: OK, and he is your role model.

P: *(Nods head yes.)*

T: So will you listen to him?

P: *(Nods head yes.)*

T: Can I hear it?

P: I forgive myself; I forgive myself for not being there for my father.

T: I really, really hope so.

P: I only have to believe it.

T: I said I hope so.

P: I know.

T: You cry for your father.

P: *(Sobs.)*

T: We can hope. You're willing to turn your father over to God.

P: *(Nods head yes.)*

T: It's hard for you to let go and let someone else look after him.

P: I will let go, I will let go.

T: You are letting go. I can see it.

P: I'll let go. He's protected.

T: How does it feel to turn your father over to God's protection?

P: At first I felt really afraid and then I started to pull back, and then I start to grab him with all I've got and pull him back.

T: I could understand that on one hand, but that would be the weak part of the ego, wouldn't it?

P: Right, I want to give him back to God.

T: Yes, and tolerate the pain of separateness.

P: Yes, I want him to be with God.

T: Because in your childhood, remember, you never learned to tolerate the pain of separateness—you were never allowed to or encouraged to. So what's it like to acknowledge the separateness?

P: It makes me feel mature. It makes me feel stronger.

T: A good feeling—you are having a good feeling about yourself.

P: Yes, it makes me feel like he taught me well, he taught me to have the strength.

T: So if you were able to send a message to your father about your current state of mind and he could receive it, what would that message be?

P: I love you; I know you're safe. Watch over me and help protect me from where you are now and help me protect myself from myself so that I can take care of my children, I can take care of my wife, I can take care of us.

T: So, in other words, you are asking him to continue to be a role model.

P: Yes, help me to be role model that he is . . . was.

T: So you feel there has been some significant psychological change in these, what did we do, six-to-eight hours of psychotherapy?

P: I don't know, Dr. Neborsky. All I can say is that it is stunning. It's almost like I feel I threw myself back and it's just such a stunning relief. I always thought that if I could understand something I could make a change. If I could understand this and reflect upon it, then I could make changes in my personality and stop and have the strength to not smoke pot, to not lash out, and to examine my anxiety and say, "OK, that's anxiety, alright."

T: And to understand its function.

P: Right.

T: I think that you understand the function now as well as anyone could.

P: I see how it punishes me.

T: Right, it's what keeps you stuck.

P: Right.

The patient returns later for a second block of therapy. Dr. Neborsky asks if their previous work together had an enduring effect. We enter this brief vignette at the beginning of the session.

P: I think recognizing the anxiety right off the bat, I think it is like any practice: the closer you are to it, the more the results last. And as you get further away from it, I guess at least initially, for me, right now, there were many fewer flare-ups with my wife over this last month.

T: It's been about that long.

P: I think the big things—the two major things for me—was beginning to understand my relationship with my mother at birth and seeing that my father was my hero and being able to . . . to relinquish . . . to let him go and to say goodbye.
T: So that really stuck with you.
P: Those two aspects of our first time together really made a difference, besides understanding and identifying the signs of anxiety.
T: And paying attention to them.
P: And paying attention to them, exactly.

During this final block of therapy the patient realized that his older brother's suicide was an act of revenge against their mother for her depression at the dropping and killing of her infant. The patient experienced his rage guilt, grief and love (forgiveness) for his self-destructive brother and left therapy with the determination to end this ongoing tragedy by loving and protecting his wife and children rather than punishing them and himself for crimes in the nursery many years ago.

At the time of this publication, the patient is a calm and sober father of two lovely twin boys.

The authors wish to express thanks to Josette ten Have-de Labije, PsyD, for her valuable insights into superego-ego processes.

BIBLIOGRAPHY

Ainsworth, M. S., Blehar, et al (1978). Patterns of Attachment: A Psychological Study of the Strange Situation. Oxford, England: Lawrence Erlbaum.

Arbib, M., (2005). The Mirror System Hypothesis. Linking Language to Theory of Mind, Interdisciples.Org/coevolution/papers/11

Bowlby, J. (1988). A secure base: Parent-child attachment and healthy human development. New York: Basic Books.

Botvinick, M., J.A.P, Bylsma, et al (2005). Viewing facial expressions of pain engages cortical areas involved in the direct experience of pain. NeuroImage, 25, 312–319.

Catmur, C.; Walsh, V. & Heyes, C. (2007), Sensorimotor learning configures the human mirror system, Current Biology 17 (17): 1527–1531.

Cheng, Y., Yang, C.Y. et al (2008). The perception of pain in others suppresses somatosensory oscillations: a magneto-encephalography study. Neuro Image, 40, 1833–1840.

Davanloo, H. (1988a). Clinical manifestations of superego pathology. Part II. The resistance of the superego and the liberation of the paralyzed ego. International Journal of Short-Term Psychotherapy,3, 1–24.

Davanloo, H. (1990). Clinical Manifestations of Superego Pathology. Unlocking the Unconscious. Chichester: Wiley.

Dinstein I., Thomas C., Behrmann M., Heeger D.J. (2008). A mirror up to nature. Curr. Biol 18 (1): R13–8.

Decety, J. (2002). Naturaliser l'empathie [Empathy naturalized]. L'Encéphale, 28, 9–20.

Decety, J., & Jackson, P.L. (2004). The functional architecture of human empathy. Behavioral and Cognitive Neuroscience Reviews, 3, 71–100.

Etzel, J.; Gazzola, V.; Keysers, C. (2008), Testing simulation theory with cross-modal multivariate classification of fMRI data, PLoS ONE 3 (11): e3690.

Fadiga, L.; Fogassi, L.; Pavesi, G.; Rizzolatti, G. (1995), Motor facilitation during action observation: a magnetic stimulation study. Journal of Neurophysiology 73 (6): 2608–2611.

Falck-Ytter, T., Gredebäck, G, von Hofsten, C (2006), Infants predict other people's action goals, Nature Neuroscience 9.

Flanagan, J. R.; Johansson, R. S. (2003), Action plans used in action observation, Nature 424 (6950): 769–771.

Fogassi, L. et al., (2005) Parietal Lobe: From Action Organization to Intention Understanding, Science308: 662–667.

Freud, S. (1923). The Ego and the Id, Hogarth, London.

Freud, A. (1936). Ego and the Mechanisms of Defenses. International University Press. London.

Gallese, V., & Goldman, A.I. (1998). Mirror neurons and the simulation theory. Trends in Cognitive Sciences, 2, 493–501.

Gallese, V.; Fadiga, L.; Fogassi, L.; Rizzolatti, G. (1996), Action recognition in the premotor cortex. Brain 119 (2): 593–609.

Gallese, V., and Goldman, A. (1998). Mirror neurons and the simulation theory of mind reading. Trends in Cognitive Sciences. 2: 493–501.

Gallese, V. (2001). The "Shared Manifold" hypothesis: from mirror neurons to empathy. Journal of Consciousness Studies, 8, 33–50.

Gazzola, V.; Keysers, C. (2009), The observation and execution of actions share motor and somatosensory voxels in all tested subjects: single-subject analyses of unsmoothed fMRI data. Cereb. Cortex 19 (6): 1239–1255.

Goldman, A. (1989). Interpretation psychologized. Mind and Language 4: 161–185.

ten Have-de Labije, J. (2009) She only wanted some understanding: Separating Ego and Superego Parts with an Extremely Anxious Woman Ad Hoc Bulletin of Short-Term Dynamic Psychotherapy.

Iacoboni, M.; Woods, R. et al (1999) Cortical Mechanisms of Human Imitation, Science 286 (5449): 2526–2528.

Karr-Morse, M., Wiley, M.S. (1997) Ghosts from the Nursery. Atlantic Monthly Press, New York.

Keysers, C., Gazzola, V (2006) Progress in Brain Research, Vol. 156.

Keysers C. and Gazzola V. (2007) Integrating simulation and theory of mind: from self to social cognition. Trends in Cognitive Sciences 11(5):194–6.

Kilner J.M., Neal A. et al (2009) Evidence of mirror neurons in human inferior frontal gyrus. J Neuroscience 29(32):10153–9.

Klein, M. (1946) Notes on some schizoid mechanisms., Int. J. Psychoanal., 27:99–110.

Lamm, C., Batson, C.D., & Decety, J. (2007). The neural substrate of human empathy: effects of perspective-taking and cognitive appraisal. Journal of Cognitive Neuroscience, 19, 42–58.

Lingnau, A; Gesierich, B; et al (2009), Asymmetric fMRI adaptation reveals no evidence for mirror neurons in humans. PNAS 106 (24): 9925–9930.

Main. M.: (2000). The organized categories of infant, child, and adult attachment: Flexible vs. inflexible attention under attachment-related stress. Journal of the American Psychoanalytic Association, 48 (4):1055–1096.

Meltzoff, A.N., & Decety, J. (2003). What imitation tells us about social cognition: A rapprochement between developmental psychology and cognitive neuroscience. The Philosophical Transactions of the Royal Society, London, 358, 491–500.

Morrison, I., Lloyd, D., di Pellegrino, G., & Roberts, N. (2004). Vicarious responses to pain in anterior cingulate cortex: is empathy a multisensory issue? Cognitive and Affective Behavioral Neuroscience, 4, 270–278.

Preston, S. D., de Waal, F.B.M. (2002) Empathy: Its ultimate and proximate bases. Behavioral and Brain Sciences, 25, 1–72.

Ramachandran, V.S. Mirror Neurons and imitation learning as the driving force behind "the great leap forward" in human evolution. Edge Foundation. 2006-11-16.

Rizzolatti, G.; Craighero, L (2004), The mirror-neuron system, Annual Review of Neuroscience 27: 169–192.

Rizzolatti, G. et al. (1996) Premotor cortex and the recognition of motor actions. Cognitive Brain Research 3 131–141.

Singer, T. et al., (2004) Science: 303, 1157.

Sommerville, J. A., & Decety, J. (2006). Weaving the fabric of social interaction: articulating developmental psychology and cognitive neuroscience in the domain of motor cognition. Psychonomic Bulletin & Review, 13, 179–200.

Sroufe, A., Egeland, et al (2005). The Development of the Person. Guilford Press.

Stevens, A. (2003) Archetype Revisited. Inner City Books, Toronto, Canada.

Théoret, H.; Pascual-L, Alvaro (2002) Language Acquisition: Do As You Hear, Current Biology, Vol. 12, No. 21, pp. R736–R737, 10–29.

van IJzendoorn, M.H., Sagi-Schwartz, A. (2008). Cross-Cultural Patterns of Attachment; Universal and Contextual Dimensions. in Cassidy, J., Shaver, P.R. Handbook of Attachment: Theory, Research and Clinical Applications. New York and London: Guilford Press. pp. 880–905.

Acknowledgments

I want to thank my daughter, Joanna Neborsky, for her dedicated efforts to make these two volumes of diverse papers into a coherent collection of writings. It would have been impossible to do it without her sharp editorial eye. In addition, her beautiful cover illustrations have made these volumes into personal treasures. I also want to thank my close friend, colleague and co-author Emanuel Peluso, whose tireless editing of my videos made many of these articles possible. Last but not least, I thank Michele Afoa, not only for her transcriptions of the later articles, but for her loyalty, reliability and efficiency, which give me the support needed to practice, teach and pursue creative activities.